SCHOOL–HOME NOTES
Promoting Children's Classroom Success

The Guilford School Practitioner Series

EDITORS

STEPHEN N. ELLIOTT, Ph.D.
University of Wisconsin—Madison

JOSEPH C. WITT, Ph.D.
Louisiana State University, Baton Rouge

Academic Skills Problems: Direct Assessment and Intervention
EDWARDS S. SHAPIRO

Curriculum-Based Measurement: Assessing Special Children
MARK R. SHINN (ED.)

Suicide Intervention in the Schools
SCOTT POLAND

Problems in Written Expression: Assessment and Remediation
SHARON BRADLEY-JOHNSON AND JUDI LUCAS LESIAK

Individual and Group Counseling in Schools
STEWART EHLY AND RICHARD DUSTIN

School–Home Notes: Promoting Children's
Classroom Success
MARY LOU KELLEY

SCHOOL–HOME NOTES
Promoting Children's Classroom Success

MARY LOU KELLEY, Ph.D.
Louisiana State University

THE GUILFORD PRESS
New York   London

© 1990 The Guilford Press
A Division of Guilford Publications, Inc.
72 Spring Street, New York, NY 10012

All rights reserved

No part of this book may be reproduced, stored in a retrieval system, or transmitted, in any form or by any means, electronic, mechanical, photocopying, microfilming, recording, or otherwise, without written permission from the Publisher.

Printed in the United States of America

This book is printed on acid-free paper.

Last digit is print number: 9 8 7 6 5 4 3 2

Library of Congress Cataloging-in-Publication Data

Kelley, Mary Lou.
    School-home notes : promoting children's classroom
success / Mary Lou Kelley.
       p.   cm.—(The Guilford school practitioner series)
    Includes bibliographical references.
    ISBN 0-89862-356-1   ISBN 0-89862-235-2 (pbk.)
    1. Home and school—United States. 2. Parent-teacher
relationships—United States. 3. Education—United States—Parent
participation. 4. Home and school—United States—Case studies.
I. Title.
LC225.3.K45   1990
371.1'03-dc20   89-49686
                                                                   CIP

To my father, Jim Kelley,
and my husband, Owen Scott.

Acknowledgments

In the course of my career many people have contributed to my knowledge of applied behavior analysis and to my development as a behavior therapist. These individuals include Lynne Embry, Donald Baer, Jon Krapfl, Trevor Stokes, and Ron Drabman. I gratefully acknowledge their impact on my career. Since taking my position on the faculty of Louisiana State University I have received valued guidance and support from many colleagues, especially Johnny Matson and Don Williamson.

My graduate students at LSU, many of whom have now successfully embarked on their own careers, have contributed greatly to my professional development and to this book. These individuals include Tim Cavell, Laura Carper, Rob Heffer, and Linda Little.

I would like to acknowledge particularly the contribution of Laura Carper to this book. Prior to the writing of the manuscript, Laura and I spent many hours discussing school–home notes in the context of actual clinical practice. Laura contributed substantially to this book, writing Chapter 2 (based on a previous chapter that we coauthored) and also the end of Chapter 3, beginning with the section on Direct Observation. Her efforts and ideas have been much appreciated throughout our personal and professional association.

I would also like to recognize the contributions of Debbie Miller and Ginger Kendall, each of whom wrote a case example that appears in Chapter 6. Linda Little assisted with the editing and with the preparation of some of the tables, and Nanette Arceneaux also made a significant contribution through her meticulous copy-editing and word processing.

Finally, I would like to recognize the contribution made by my husband, Owen Scott. Through conceptual, methodological, and editorial input, as well as emotional support, he makes his presence felt in my professional work. Owen is more than just a footnote in my life.

Mary Lou Kelley
Louisiana State University

Contents

Chapter 1. Introduction   1

    Case Example   2
    Common Obstacles to Parent–Teacher
      Communication   3
    School–Home Notes   4

Chapter 2. Literature Review: The Efficacy of
      School–Home Notes   10

    History   10
    Factors Influencing the Efficacy of School–Home
      Notes   11
    Summary   23

Chapter 3. Assessment of School and Home
      Functioning   25

    Behavioral Assessment   25
    Additional Assessment Considerations   33
    Assessment Procedures   45
    Summary   59
    Appendix 3.1 Child Intake Form for Use in a
      Parent Interview   60

Chapter 4. Developing and Using School–Home
      Notes   64

    Setting the Stage   65
    Designing the School–Home Note Program   75
    Negotiating Behavior Change Contracts   84
    Implementing the Program   92
    Summary   111

Appendix 4.1   A Handout for Parents and
    Teachers on School–Home Notes   115
Appendix 4.2   Sample School–Home Notes   119
Appendix 4.3   School–Home Note Contract and
    Record Form   127
Appendix 4.4   A Handout for Parents on Star
    Charts   131

Chapter 5.   Special Applications of School–Home
    Notes   133

Response Cost   133
Overcorrection   140
Uses of School–Home Notes with Special
    Populations   145
Adolescents   148
Summary and Concluding Remarks   150
Appendix 5.1   A Handout for Parents and
    Teachers on the General Use of Response Cost   152
Appendix 5.2   School–Home Notes that Include
    a Response Cost Component   155

Chapter 6.   Case Illustrations   158

Martin   158
Jim   163
Lauren   168
Bill   172
Steve   176

References   182
Index   192

1

Introduction

Parent involvement in the schools has long been heralded as an important ingredient in children's academic success. In fact, legal and ethical dictates demand parent participation in planning and executing children's educational goals and programs. For example, Public Law 94-142 and its recent amendment for preschoolers (i.e., P.L. 99-457) require collaboration between parents and schools in the delivery of special education services. Parents and teachers typically appreciate each other's influence and view open dialogue as essential to promoting children's optimal functioning. It is generally assumed that establishing complementary expectations at home and school will foster children's development. Children are presented with a united front when parents and teachers work together to teach new skills and discourage inappropriate behavior. Children realize that they cannot manipulate one set of adults against the other, and often learn to adhere to rules. On the other hand, when problems occur in one environment, we assume that behavior will be affected in the other. For example, children often function poorly at school when their parents are excessively punitive, provide too little structure, or are experiencing serious marital or substance abuse problems. Children who are teased by their peers at school or who experience difficulty learning may express their distress through negative, irritable behavior at home.

Teachers and parents may communicate well and solve minor problems quickly and easily. A thoughtful teacher may telephone a parent when a problem arises to allow the parents an opportunity to discuss the situation with their child. Parents and teachers may develop methods of solving problems such as inconsistent homework completion by writing notes to each other on a frequent basis.

Although parent–teacher communication sometimes produces successful outcomes, these collaborative efforts often seem to complicate children's poor classroom adjustment. Sometimes communication efforts produce a great deal of ineffective or negative interaction between school and home, and/or fail to improve children's problem behavior. These problems rarely are due to adults' lack of interest in helping the problem child. Therefore, what factors prevent parents and teachers from cooperatively and effectively promoting children's academic success and overall adjustment? In part, poor communication may be due to the fact that formal methods of beginning and maintaining communication have not been established in most school systems. Schools often are not accustomed to including parents in problem-solving efforts. As the following case example illustrates, many misunderstandings and obstacles to effective problem solving can occur when parents and teachers attempt to work together to remediate children's classroom behavior problems.

CASE EXAMPLE

Timothy is a 10-year-old boy who frequently refuses to complete his classwork. Instead, he daydreams, walks around the room, or talks to other children. When he does attempt to complete his work, he often hurries through the assignment and makes careless errors. Because Timothy has demonstrated an ability to do the required work, his problems do not appear to be due to a lack of skill, but to other factors. Timothy's teacher, Mrs. Smith, reports having tried numerous classroom interventions such as making Timothy stay in from recess to do his work, praising Timothy when he completes his work, and sending notes home that list the assignments he needs to finish. Mrs. Smith is convinced that the parents are not doing all that they can do to improve Timothy's school behavior. She admits being frustrated with the situation and states, "It's to the point where I just let him sit there as long as he is not bothering anyone else."

Timothy's parents, Mr. and Mrs. Warren, are equally frustrated. They report that Timothy is a bright child who has always done well in school. The parents believe that they have attempted to solve Timothy's problems, but without success. The Warrens frequently talk to Timothy about his schoolwork and have forbidden him to watch TV or ride his bike until his grades improve. Even spanking has not had any apparent effect. The Warrens spend about 2 hours each evening working with Timothy on his homework. However, they admit, "We cannot spend our entire evening with him any more. We have two other children who also need our attention. This problem is really interfering with our family life." The Warrens report that the only time they hear from the teacher is when Timothy is misbehaving. They feel that if Mrs. Smith were a better, more interested teacher, Timothy would be performing satisfactorily in school.

COMMON OBSTACLES TO PARENT–TEACHER COMMUNICATION

The preceding case example illustrates some of the problems that can occur when children fail to perform adequately in school. It is common, for example, for teachers and parents to communicate ineffectively and to blame each other for creating or maintaining children's academic problems. Parents often feel that there is little they can do beyond taking away privileges or enforcing an established time for homework; they simply are not present in the school environment where problems occur. Feedback to parents regarding children's academic and social performance is often intermittent and negative. Parents complain that they only hear about the negative things their children do. Often, by the time they do obtain such a report, the problem is relatively long-standing. Given parents' inability to provide frequent, immediate consequences in a contingent manner, it is understandable that they may blame teachers for failing to remediate their children's classroom behavior problems. It is easy to see how a frustrated parent may assume that a teacher's deficiencies or flaws are responsible for a child's problems.

Teachers may counter these criticisms by reminding parents that they are overworked and responsible for educating a large number of children. True, it is unreasonable to expect teachers to employ an intervention that is time-consuming; such a procedure may unfairly limit the time available for teaching or working with other students. Teachers may also remind parents that they are in a profession with few financial incentives; this implies that they sincerely care about their students' classroom adjustment. Classroom teachers may conclude that because they do not have problems with all their students, the problems exhibited by a specific child reflect deficits in parenting. Likewise, teachers may attribute a child's problems to external factors such as the child's temperament, familial dysfunction, or parental stress. Finally, it is common for teachers to encounter defensive, apparently unmotivated parents who would rather blame the school system or the teacher than wholeheartedly attempt to solve their children's problems.

Fortunately, more often than not parents and teachers sincerely want a problem child to succeed in the classroom. Both parties typically are willing to work toward remediating children's classroom deficits. The constraints that limit parents' and teachers' ability to employ effective interventions, however, are real; these limitations must be addressed if recommended treatments are to be used with integrity and in ways that produce minimal negative side effects. Workable treatments must be not only effective, but minimally obtrusive, minimally time-consuming, and not preferential to a single child.

Numerous ways exist in which parents and teachers can work together in a more positive, collaborative manner. In most schools, parents can attend regularly scheduled conferences, participate in classroom activities, and inquire periodically about their child's performance. Teachers can facilitate communication and collaboration by routinely conducting conferences, informing parents about the child's performance, and sending home papers on classroom activities.

Many times, these routine procedures are adequate for problem solving and maintaining positive parent-teacher relationships. However, in cases such as Timothy's, more formally developed and administered treatments are often necessary.

SCHOOL–HOME NOTES

One viable intervention that minimizes the time required of teachers while providing parents with increased opportunities to give effective consequences is a "school–home note" or "daily report card." The procedure requires that parents and teachers work together toward alleviating children's classroom behavior problems. Use of school–home notes requires teachers to evaluate children's behavior on a daily basis and parents to deliver consequences based on each evaluation. Children generally are responsible for bringing the notes home. Like other behavioral interventions, school–home notes are most effective when they focus on changing socially valid, objectively defined behavior and prompt the delivery of salient, immediate, and frequent positive consequences contingent on satisfactory behavior.

In the example above, Mrs. Smith and the Warrens may meet with a consultant to select important target behaviors. In Timothy's case, work completion is a likely choice; Timothy's lack of productivity affects his academic skill acquisition and causes significant problems at home due to excessive homework. Figure 1.1 shows the school–home note that may be used to improve Timothy's work completion. As shown in the figure, Mrs. Smith indicates the percentage of each

SCHOOL–HOME NOTE

Name _____ Timothy _____   **Date** _____

CLASS: _____ Reading _____

Percentage of work
   completed correctly   NA 0 25 50 75   90 or above
Behaved cooperatively before
   and during class period   Yes So-so No

Comments:

_____

CLASS: _____ Math _____

Percentage of work
   completed correctly   NA 0 25 50 75   90 or above
Behaved cooperatively before
   and during class period   Yes So-so No

Comments:

_____

CLASS: _____ Spelling _____

Percentage of work
   completed correctly   NA 0 25 50 75   90 or above
Behaved cooperatively before
   and during class period   Yes So-so No

Comments:

_____

CLASS: _____ Handwriting _____

Percentage of work
   completed correctly   NA 0 25 50 75   90 or above
Behaved cooperatively before
   and during class period   Yes So-so No

Comments:

_____

CLASS: _____ Language _____

Percentage of work
   completed correctly   NA 0 25 50 75   90 or above
Behaved cooperatively before
   and during class period   Yes So-so No

Comments:

_____

(cont.)

FIGURE 1.1. Sample school–home note for use with Timothy.

SCHOOL–HOME NOTE *(continued)*

CLASS: _____Science_____

Percentage of work
    completed correctly   NA   0   25   50   75   90 or above
Behaved cooperatively before
    and during class period   Yes So-so No

Comments:

_____

Parent Comments:
Consequences provided last night:_____

_____

_____

_____

Questions/comments:_____

_____

_____

_____

class assignment correctly completed by Timothy on a given day. She can calculate this quickly after reviewing his work, without actually grading all of it. For example, when Mrs. Smith collects the papers or reviews the children's notebooks to assess their progress, she can estimate the number of problems or items completed and "spot-check" for accuracy. In all likelihood, the system will increase Mrs. Smith's monitoring of Timothy's work completion rates. This increased monitoring will prompt her to praise Timothy more often and provide him with additional feedback. Although Timothy is responsible for obtaining the evaluation from his teacher and presenting it to his parents, initially they should prompt him to do so.

The Warrens, in turn, provide Timothy with privileges when he completes a predetermined amount of classwork. The amount of classwork initially required of Timothy to obtain his privileges should be reasonable and based on the amount completed prior to the introduction of the school–home note system. If Timothy very frequently achieves criterion, the amount of correctly completed classwork required is increased over time. The privileges earned by Timothy may include readily available, daily rewards, such as watching TV in the evening or a later bedtime. Larger rewards, such as lunch at McDonald's or a special weekend activity with Dad, may be provided for consistently good performance during the previous week. Mr. and Mrs. Warren can provide Mrs. Smith with feedback or ask questions in the "parent comments" section of the note.

Although the assessment and treatment of many children with academic or classroom behavior problems are not as straightforward as in Timothy's case, school–home notes are useful in almost any situation where parent involvement might serve a therapeutic function. For example, assessment of Timothy's poor academic productivity may reveal skill deficits requiring tutoring in phonics or specific mathematic skills. Often, however, skill acquisition is enhanced through the use of incentive systems such as school–home notes (Schumaker, Hovell, & Sherman, 1977); thus, the presence of skill deficits or other contributory problems does not preclude the value of daily feedback to parents.

Advantages of School–Home Notes

As illustrated in the case example, the use of school–home notes has numerous advantages over other interventions for modifying children's classroom behavior (Atkeson & Forehand, 1979; Kelley & Carper, 1988). The potential benefits include the following:

1. The procedure requires parents and teachers to define target behavior and treatment goals jointly. This collaboration focuses on problem solving rather than on labeling the "problem causer."

2. Administration of the procedure requires the combined effort of parents and teachers. Thus, neither party is burdened with the sole responsibility for problem solving.

3. School–home notes provide parents with very frequent feedback and emphasize positive rather than negative behavior. Consequently, communication between teachers and parents often improves as both parties increase their focus on what the child does well and how the child is improving.

4. Students often appreciate the added feedback and established performance criteria associated with the use of school–home notes. Students often feel a greater sense of control over their situation than they do when feedback is intermittent and negative.

5. Because parents, rather than teachers, are responsible for providing consequences, use of the procedure requires only minimal teacher time. Therefore, teachers may be more likely to employ the procedure with integrity and to view the intervention as acceptable.

6. It is not necessary for teachers to alter their teaching routines substantially when employing daily report cards. They simply eval-

uate students' behavior in a systematic manner and provide this information to parents.

7. Home-based reinforcement programs do not produce many of the problems associated with in-class reinforcement. In particular, the procedure addresses teachers' concerns over the inequity of giving special rewards to only a few students.

8. Parents often have access to and control over a wider variety of children's reinforcers than do teachers. Thus, the procedure may be more effective because rewards in the home are more salient than those available from teachers.

9. As most school–home note procedures emphasize positive behavior, children often are provided with increased parental praise and attention. This not only may improve classroom behavior, but may also foster children's self-esteem and self-efficacy.

10. Reinforcers are provided at the end of the school day. This delayed reinforcement may enhance generalization of treatment by teaching children to behave appropriately in the absence of immediate gratification.

Purpose of This Book

Like many behavioral interventions, school–home notes are simple in concept. However, as is true of other behavior modification programs, many professional skills are required to develop and administer an effective school–home note program. The consultant who offers the procedure to parents and teachers as a medium for improving students' classroom behavior must be a skilled mediator, problem solver, and behavior analyst. He or she must be effective at working with both parents and teachers. For example, the consultant should be familiar with the assessment of maternal and familial dysfunction, because problems in these areas may interfere with school performance. He or she should be skilled in interviewing teachers and eliciting their cooperation. The consultant also must be able to determine when a school–home note is unlikely to be effective because of environmental obstacles, or inappropriate because of the nature of the child's skill deficits.

Although this book is not intended to be a crash course in behavioral techniques, Chapter 3 is devoted to the assessment of classroom and home environments in order to provide a context for the appropriate use of incentive systems in general and daily report cards in particular. The primary purposes of the volume, however, are to provide professionals with the following:

- A critical appraisal of the relevant literature on parent- and teacher-managed contingency systems
- Practical information on designing and implementing effective school–home notes and other family-based interventions that facilitate appropriate classroom adjustment
- Guidelines for determining when the procedures are appropriate to use alone or in combination with other interventions
- A variety of handouts, sample school–home notes, and illustrative case examples

2

Literature Review: The Efficacy of School–Home Notes

LAURA CARPER
MARY LOU KELLEY

The purpose of this chapter is to acquaint the reader with the literature supporting the use of school–home notes or home-based reinforcement. We first review the history leading to this type of approach, and then discuss research studies that have investigated the effects of school–home notes on students' classroom behavior. Specifically, the chapter reviews the various types of parent–teacher communication procedures employed in the literature, as well as the wide range of subjects, target behaviors, and consequences included in such programs. The varying degree of parent and teacher involvement in the development and administration of the procedure is discussed as well. Finally, issues relevant to program efficacy and social validity are presented.

HISTORY

Behavior therapists have become increasingly reliant on parents and teachers to employ interventions for changing children's behavior. The use of adults as contingency managers has proven to be both an efficient and an effective method of remediating children's behavior problems.

Parent training is an important example of this trend. The approach involves teaching parents skills for improving their children's behavior (Berkowitz & Graziano, 1972; Mash, Hamerlynck, & Handy,

1976; Moreland, Schwebel, Beck, & Wells, 1982; O'Dell, 1974; Reisinger, Ora, & Frangia, 1976). Parents are commonly taught to reduce their children's misbehavior through their use of clear instructions and effective, consistent consequences. Use of such techniques as differential attention, time out, and reward procedures have proven effective in reducing such problems as noncompliance (Bernal, Klinnert, & Schultz, 1980; Forehand & King, 1977), stealing (Stumphauzer, 1976), and verbal and physical aggression (Patterson, Chamberlain, & Reid, 1982; Wahler & Fox, 1980).

In the classroom, teachers also have been taught to change children's behavior through the use of contingency management techniques. These techniques have included time out (Porterfield, Herbert-Jackson, & Risley, 1976), praise and ignoring (McAllister, Stachowiak, Baer, & Conderman, 1969), and overcorrection (Foxx & Jones, 1978), as well as reward and response cost procedures (Long & Williams, 1973). Teachers' use of contingency management techniques, like that of parents, has proven effective with a variety of target behaviors. Academic behaviors such as staying on task, studying, and completing assignments have increased with the use of contingency management techniques. Similarly, classroom behavior problems such as fighting and talking out of turn have been reduced successfully through teachers' use of behavioral interventions. These interventions have been applied to both entire classrooms of students and individual children.

Collaboration between parents and teachers for the purpose of promoting children's competent functioning in the classroom has increased in recent years. In part, this increased collaboration is due to the dictates of P.L. 94-142, which emphasizes teachers' legal and professional obligation to include parents in the educational process. In addition, professionals working with children have noted the benefits of increased communication between parents and teachers (Guidubaldi, 1982). The effect of this increased awareness has been the creation and utilization of home-based reinforcement systems for modifying children's classroom behavior. These programs have provided parents with information about their child's classroom performance, so that parents may assist in improving academic and behavioral problems.

FACTORS INFLUENCING THE EFFICACY OF SCHOOL–HOME NOTES

Quality and Specificity of Parent–Teacher Communication

To be effective, school–home notes should provide parents with enough information about the child's classroom performance that appropriate consequences can be delivered at home (Broughton, Barton, & Owen, 1981). Because this communication is so important, several key features have been included across studies. For example, target behaviors are usually defined by the teacher (or with his or her input) and are evaluated consistently across school days. In most cases, the teacher evaluates whether or not the child performed the relevant target behaviors. Parents are usually provided with this information on a daily basis. In all studies reviewed, both parents and children were familiar with the purpose of the procedure and the consequences for positive or negative performance. Finally, in most cases, the school–home note system is similar to a token economy, in that children contingently earn positive feedback that represents rewards to be received at a later time (Broughton et al., 1981).

The criteria used by teachers to evaluate classroom performance have varied considerably. In several studies, feedback provided to parents was rather general, although the evaluation criteria used by teachers were quite specific. For example, Karraker (1972) provided parents with global descriptions of children's behavior, yet the criteria used by teachers were very specific: A satisfactory evaluation was earned when a child increased or maintained either his or her class rank in mathematics or the percentage of problems completed correctly. Similarly, the criteria for the "Brag Sheet" used in a study by Ayllon, Garber, and Pisor (1975) were operationally defined as no more than two disruptions within a 15-minute block of time; however, parents were provided only with nonspecific letters on days when their children exhibited low levels of disruptive behavior. In contrast to these studies, Schumaker et al. (1977) required teachers to evaluate students' performance of an array of responses although the criteria for determining whether or not the behaviors occurred were not specified precisely.

In several studies, teachers operationalized the evaluation criteria as well as provided parents with specific feedback (Blechman, Kotanchik, & Taylor, 1981; Budd, Leibowitz, Riner, Mindell, & Goldfarb, 1981; Lahey et al., 1977). For example, Blechman, Kotanchik, and Taylor (1981) noted improved academic performance when parents were provided with objective feedback. In this study, prior to the initiation of the note procedure, each student and a parent met individually with the teacher to review the student's baseline performance and to negotiate a specific contract. The procedure in this study included objective evaluation criteria and detailed feedback, as well as assistance to parents in delineating the specific criteria for earning rewards.

Whether teachers evaluate children according to operationally defined criteria or provide parents with detailed feedback does not appear to be systematically related to treatment outcome. Although school–home notes have been found effective in most studies, regardless of the specificity of the performance criteria, it is very likely that some level of objectivity and detail is necessary for the procedure to be effective. In addition, treatment outcome may be differentially affected by the level of detail contained in the note (Broughton et al., 1981). It is possible that the importance of specificity and objectivity in teacher ratings and communication to parents may be related to student characteristics, such as age or type of behavior problem, as well as to the parents' education level or parenting skills. Clearly, research is needed that systematically manipulates the objectivity of performance criteria and the quality of information contained in the school–home note.

The comprehensiveness of home-based contingency programs has varied widely. For instance, work accuracy in one subject area has often been the only dependent measure (Blechman, Kotanchik, & Taylor, 1981; Blechman, Taylor, & Schrader, 1981; Karraker, 1972). In contrast, several studies have evaluated children's behavior throughout the entire school day (e.g., Budd et al., 1981; Schumaker et al., 1977). Budd et al. (1981) employed a comprehensive school–home note procedure with preschool and kindergarten-age children. The school day was divided into 12 intervals, during each of which the children could earn a sticker if they had not engaged in a target response. Thus, although the intervention encompassed behavior performed throughout the day, the children were given many opportunities to achieve small goals.

The majority of school–home note interventions sought to change the frequency of a single behavior during a portion of the day. In some instances, it appeared that only a single behavior deficit or excess existed; commonly, however, children display more pervasive behavior problems that are not limited in occurrence to a specific academic period or subject. Consequently, logistical and methodological issues involved in the comprehensive use of a school–home note procedure have not been adequately addressed. For example, broadening the comprehensiveness of the school–home note to include children's behavior throughout the day may require the selection of target behaviors that are more easily monitored by teachers than are those typically reported in the literature.

Teachers usually evaluate students on a daily basis, although in several studies parents were provided with notes only on days when the children behaved satisfactorily. Ayllon, Garber, and Pisor (1975) gave parents a "good behavior letter" on days when their children engaged in low levels of disruptiveness, and did not provide feedback when the children behaved in an unsatisfactory way. Parents were informed, however, that the absence of a note indicated that their children were demonstrating severe behavior problems, and were told to reprimand accordingly. Similarly, Lahey et al. (1977) rewarded children with "Brag Sheets" when they met defined criteria, and Blechman and colleagues (Blechman, Kotanchik, & Taylor, 1981; Blechman, Taylor, & Schrader, 1981) provided congratulatory letters to bring home.

In the studies reviewed, rationales for providing daily reports as opposed to feedback only when children behave satisfactorily have typically not been provided. It is possible that giving only positive feedback may decrease the likelihood that children will be severely punished at home for poor performance (Lahey et al., 1977). The procedure may also result in greater teacher satisfaction, because the teacher probably completes fewer notes. However, providing parents with only positive evaluations is really partial communication; it may prevent parents from fully monitoring, and thus consistently providing consequences for, their children's behavior. Whether the two forms of feedback are differentially effective or socially valid can only be speculated upon, as empirical evaluations addressing the issue have not been conducted.

Age and Problems of Students

Home-based reinforcement techniques have resulted in improved classroom behavior of children of many ages. School-home notes have been implemented to improve the classroom conduct and academic performance of kindergarteners (Budd et al., 1981), elementary-age children (Imber, Imber, & Rothstein, 1979; Saudargas, Madsen, & Scott, 1977; Todd, Scott, Bostow, & Alexander, 1976), and junior high and high school students (Alexander, Corbett, & Smigel, 1976; Heaton, Safer, Allen, Spinnato, & Prumo, 1976; Schumaker et al., 1977). Most studies have been conducted with younger children; relatively few studies have employed adolescents as subjects. The implementation of school–home notes with adolescents has typically involved students residing in group homes or institutional settings.

Home-based reinforcement systems have been used with students varying in their baseline performance levels. Subjects in several studies were not identified as having any specific behavioral or academic problems (Dougherty & Dougherty, 1977; Lahey et al., 1977; Saudargas et al., 1977). These studies employed school–home notes with entire classrooms of children and were successful in obtaining overall academic improvement. Home-based reinforcement systems have also been used to remediate specific problems, such as excessive disruptiveness (Budd et al., 1981; Heaton et al., 1976) or poor academic performance (Anesko & O'Leary, 1983; Imber et al., 1979). Studies employing students with behavior problems have found school–home notes to be effective with entire classrooms of children as well as with individual students.

Target Behaviors

Teachers and parents have modified a wide range of classroom behaviors through their use of school–home notes (Broughton et al., 1981). For example, a variety of disruptive behaviors have been reduced through the use of home-based reinforcement programs, such as talking out during class (Dougherty & Dougherty, 1977), inappropriate behavior during naptime (Lahey et al., 1977), and classroom rule violations.

Many studies using school–home notes have centered on academic behaviors. Some researchers have targeted academic products or outcomes, such as the amount or quality of completed classwork (Blechman, Taylor, & Schrader, 1981; Dougherty & Dougherty, 1977; Imber et al, 1979; Saudargas et al., 1977). Others have found improvement in process variables, such as staying on task (Coleman, 1973) or studying (Bailey, Wolf, & Phillips, 1970).

In a few studies, the effects of targeting academic process versus outcome variables have been compared; however, considerable support exists for targeting the latter. Some researchers suggest that outcome variables such as work completion and accuracy are the goals for any student and should therefore be the variables targeted for change (Winett & Winkler, 1972). Parents and teachers generally concur about the value of academic productivity; however, considerable disagreement may exist over what constitutes appropriate classroom conduct. Academic outcomes, such as percentage of work completed, can be monitored quickly and objectively by teachers. Academic behaviors are relatively easy for parents to interpret; this may facilitate both teacher involvement and consistent delivery of consequence by parents. Finally, research has shown that when children are rewarded for increased academic productivity, improvements in classroom conduct occur simultaneously (Ayllon, Layman, & Kandel, 1975; Kirby & Shields, 1972). After all, few children can complete all their work accurately and have time to misbehave. In contrast, researchers targeting disruptiveness have not always found simultaneous improvements in academic performance (Ferritor, Buckholdt, Hamblin, & Smith, 1972; Wagner & Guyer, 1971).

A great deal of variability exists in the specificity of target responses. Information provided to parents from teachers has ranged from very specific to very global feedback. For example, Karraker (1972) provided parents with a daily report card that indicated whether the child had exhibited satisfactory performance in mathematics. In contrast, Schumaker et al. (1977) provided very specific feedback regarding seventh-grade students' performance of 13 academic and social behaviors.

Consequences

The goals in any contingency management system are to reinforce appropriate behavior (so as to increase its frequency) and to ignore or punish inappropriate or unacceptable behavior (so as to decrease its frequency). Thus, with the school–home note system, appropriate parental consequences are perhaps the most important aspect of the procedure. In the research literature, consequences have included response cost, praise, tangible rewards, and various combinations of these procedures. Consequences have been offered to children contingent on both satisfactory and unsatisfactory notes. Although most studies included parental praise as a component, several investigators used praise as the only consequence for appropriate behavior in the classroom (Doughtery & Doughtery, 1977; Lahey et al., 1977). In these studies, parents were instructed to praise their children contingent on satisfactory school reports. Both of these studies were conducted with entire classrooms of children exhibiting no serious behavior problems. Lahey et al. (1977) recommended that parents praise their children for satisfactory performance according to the school–home note and that they avoid punishing poor performance. The procedure used in these studies was effective in increasing students' appropriate behavior.

In another study, the effects of praise alone were compared with those of praise plus privileges on the classroom behavior and academic performance of an adolescent boy (Schumaker et al., 1977). It was found that praise alone was ineffective. In fact, on most days during the praise-only condition, the subject did not bring the card home. However, with the introduction of praise and privileges, the student's classwork and adherence to classroom rules improved substantially.

Other investigators have combined praise with tangible rewards for good behavior at school (Alexander et al., 1976; Blechman, Taylor, & Schrader, 1981). Many rewards have been used, including allowances, later bedtime, and activity reinforcers (e.g., bike riding and TV time). In a study by MacDonald, Gallimore, and MacDonald (1970), school counselors contacted adults who controlled the reinforcers of six frequently truant adolescents. The counselors then negotiated "deals" between the students and the adults, such that reinforcers were contingent on school attendance. An interesting aspect of this study was that the adults were not always the students' parents; in one case, the adult was a pool hall proprietor who controlled access to the pool hall. The intervention was generally effective in increasing students' attendance.

Heaton et al. (1976) conducted a study using reinforcers from both home and school. In this study, classroom points and teacher praise were provided contingent on in-class behavior. Attractive afternoon activities at school, as well as home rewards, were contingent on a specified number of points. The combination of consequences was effective in increasing classroom working behavior.

The effects of group versus individual consequences on adolescents' class attendance were compared by Alexander et al. (1976). They found that the group consequences (which were delivered only if all members of the group attended all classes) were more effective than individual consequences in increasing class attendance.

Several investigators have compared school-based with home-based contingency systems. Ayllon, Garber, and Pisor (1975), for example, found that school-based reinforcement was only temporarily effective in modifying academic and disruptive behavior in a highly disruptive classroom. However, a "Good Behavior" letter with home rewards was more effective in reducing disruptive behavior. Karraker (1972) compared a performance feedback condition with a home reward condition in which rewards were given for satisfactory school performance. The results of this study indicated that academic productivity increased only when students were provided with home rewards. Similarly, Imber et al. (1979) found that home notes plus teacher praise were more effective than teacher praise alone.

Finally, Budd et al. (1981) compared the relative effects of three different types of consequences on students' disruptive behavior. The consequences included (1) stickers and teacher praise, (2) home rewards based on stickers earned at school, and (3) school and home rewards based on low levels of class disruptiveness. The subjects in this study were three groups of six children. The results obtained with two of the groups revealed that home rewards produced a significant decrease in disruptive behavior. These positive results were not found when stickers and teacher praise alone were employed.

In several studies, response cost procedures have been used to increase appropriate classroom behavior. For example, Bailey et al. (1970) implemented a procedure whereby students earned extra privileges at home for satisfactory classroom behavior. In this study, students lost privileges contingent on unsatisfactory notes. Similarly, Todd et al. (1976) provided a response cost in the form of a 1-day suspension from school following three undesirable daily report cards. Finally, students in the study by Ayllon, Garber, and Pisor (1975) earned and lost points contingent on behavior in the classroom.

In the study by Saudargas et al. (1977), parents were not told to provide any home contingencies based on a school–home note. No requirements were instituted to insure that the children's parents received or read the cards; therefore, it is uncertain whether the children received any parental feedback. Nevertheless, the intervention resulted in increased classwork completion.

In conclusion, research indicates that school–home notes may be more effective than school reward interventions. Studies comparing school rewards with home rewards found that home rewards produced greater changes in students' behavior. In addition, although praise should always be paired with rewards, praise alone does not seem to be a particularly potent reinforcer. This appears to be especially true for very disruptive children (Schumaker et al., 1977).

One shortcoming of the research on school–home notes has been the lack of evaluation of parents' appropriate delivery of consequences. Rarely do researchers report data on parent consequences. In the study by Budd et al. (1981), parents were asked to record consequences on the back of the report card and return it to school; however, this study is clearly the exception to the rule. More research is needed that evaluates the consistency with which home consequences are given.

Parent Involvement and Training

When parents are taught behavior management techniques for use in the home, they often learn a variety of skills. Typically, parents are taught to identify target behaviors, to monitor these behaviors, and to use a number of behavior change techniques (e.g., time out and reward procedures). However, because school–home notes are designed to modify behavior that occurs in the classroom, parents are often required only to provide consequences based on teachers' feedback. Parents' role in administering the school–home note system is often negligible, compared to their involvement in purely home-based contingency systems.

In numerous studies, school–home notes have been used successfully after only minimal contact with, or training of, the parents.

Several investigators simply provided parents with a letter explaining the purpose of the procedure and specific strategies for providing consequences at home (Dougherty & Dougherty, 1977; Karraker, 1972; Lahey et al., 1977; Saudargas et al., 1977). Lahey et al. (1977) provided parents with a letter instructing them to praise satisfactory performance but to avoid punishing their children. Even though the contact with parents in this study was minimal, the procedure was effective at improving kindergarteners' behavior during naptime. Other investigators have implemented the school–home note procedures successfully with only a moderate amount of parent training (Ayllon, Garber, & Pisor, 1975; Blechman, Kotanchik, & Taylor, 1981; Budd et al., 1981). Ayllon, Garber, and Pisor (1975), for example, reduced the disruptive behavior of 23 boys with a successful school–home note procedure. In this study, the parents were provided with a single 2-hour training session, which focused on teaching parents to praise and deliver appropriate consequences.

Researchers have also provided parents with relatively extensive training with effective consequences (Bailey et al., 1970; Blechman, Taylor, & Schrader, 1981; Schumaker et al., 1977). For example, parents of adolescent boys were provided weekly training sessions on the administration of a relatively complex school–home token economy system (Schumaker et al., 1977).

Two studies assessed the influence of the amount and type of parent training on note effectiveness. Karraker (1972) trained parents of second-graders in the use of school–home notes through either a descriptive letter, a 15-minute conference, or two 1-hour training sessions. Regardless of training condition, all parents were told to provide positive consequences when their children performed satisfactorily and to avoid commenting when notes were unsatisfactory. The results indicated that all training methods were effective in increasing the children's mathematics performance. However, because of the small number of children in each condition and the variability of baseline performance, differential treatment effects could not be ascertained.

Blechman, Taylor, and Schrader (1981) compared two parent training programs for use with daily reports from teachers. The subjects were elementary school students from 17 classrooms who performed inconsistently in mathematics. The students were assigned randomly to one of two treatment conditions or to an untreated control condition. The children in both groups received a "Good News Note" on days when their mathematics performance was satisfactory. However, parents of children in one treatment group were sent a letter explaining the purpose of the note and ways to reward satisfactory performance. Children and parents assigned to the alternate treatment were taught to negotiate a contingency contract in a family problem-solving session and were telephoned weekly to monitor contract compliance. Although both treatments decreased classwork variability compared to the control condition, children in the family problem-solving condition completed their work more accurately than did children in the letter-only condition. In addition, only the children who received the family problem-solving treatment demonstrated response maintenance on days in which the treatment was briefly withdrawn.

In summary, significant improvements in children's classroom behavior have occurred when parents are provided with only minimal instruction in the use of school–home notes. However, with the exception of Blechman, Taylor, and Schrader (1981), researchers who supplied parents with only brief written instructions employed the procedure with entire classrooms of elementary school children whose academic and classroom behavior were generally not problematic. Thus, it is unclear whether parents of older children who exhibit behavior problems would be sufficiently trained to implement the school–home note procedure if provided only with brief written instructions.

Teacher Involvement and Training

The degree to which teachers are involved in developing the school–home note and procedures has been quite variable. For example, the teachers in Schumaker et al. (1977) monitored a variety of behaviors for each student, including whether or not he or she came to class on time, brought supplies, remained seated, talked inappropriately, followed directions, and paid attention. By contrast, Doughtery and Doughtery (1977) had the teacher record only homework completion and talking without permission. In the majority of studies, teachers have been required to monitor some aspect of their students' behavior. Some researchers have provided observers to monitor classroom behavior, so that teachers were required only to complete the report card each day (Bailey et al., 1970). Few researchers have collected reliability data on teachers' monitoring of classroom behavior; however, the researchers who have calculated teachers' reliability with observers (Budd et al., 1970; Lahey et al., 1977) have generally found that teachers are reliable in their monitoring.

The use of observers certainly is more convenient for teachers; however, it would seem that in the interest of generalizability, home-based reinforcement programs should be designed so that the procedures can be assumed completely by the teacher when the experimenter leaves. In addition, the ease of monitoring and amount of time involved are important to teachers. Witt, Martens, and Elliott (1984) found that teachers view interventions requiring little teacher time as more acceptable, and therefore may be more likely to implement the simpler interventions with integrity. In addition, Broughton et al. (1981) noted that complex monitoring and observation systems may be important for research but sometimes impractical for the teacher. An objective yet simple system is probably best for clinical application.

Most investigators did not discuss any aspect of teacher training. Although researchers generally described teachers' duties in implementing the school–home note system, they did not report on how teachers were acquainted with the intervention. Only a few authors have addressed the topic of teacher training. For example, Schumaker et al. (1977) and Todd et al. (1976) held conferences with teachers to draw up the rules for school–home notes. Dougherty and Dougherty (1977) provided teachers with written instructions on rating target behaviors. Lahey et al. (1977) provided teachers with instructions on how to fill out the daily report card; these teachers were also instructed to be positive when presenting the cards. Finally, although Saudargas et al. (1977) did not discuss specific teacher training procedures, they did report that the teachers involved in their study had received previous training in the use of behavioral techniques.

In summary, researchers may have provided adequate training for their teachers, but many have not included a description of training techniques. Given that teacher training is such an important part of the home-based reinforcement system, more attention should be given to the description of the training techniques.

Maintenance of Behavior Change

Several authors have noted the importance of employing treatment maintenance techniques in the use of home-based reinforcement (Atkeson & Forehand, 1979; Broughton et al., 1981). In spite of this emphasis, few investigators have addressed issues of treatment maintenance and fading. Lahey (cited in Gresham & Lemanek, 1987) has recommended a specific fading procedure, whereby daily reports are replaced by weekly cards and then phased out completely. Other studies have used this fading technique, although data on its effectiveness are not typically provided. Dougherty and Dougherty (1977) faded daily cards to cards describing a full week's performance.

Bailey et al. (1970) faded daily cards to biweekly ones. Schumaker et al. (1977) recommended a fading procedure in which the student would carry a shortened version of the daily report card; however, their procedure was not implemented.

Some authors have briefly discussed informal maintenance procedures. For instance, Imber et al. (1979) used praise cards "intermittently" after the study was completed. The authors reported that the procedure effectively maintained student performance, although no data were reported. Because follow-up data were collected in few studies, it is difficult to assess the long-term success of school–home notes. Atkeson and Forehand (1979) noted in their review of home-based reinforcement programs that only 16% of the studies they reviewed included follow-up data. It is also difficult to examine the issue of response maintenance because most studies concluded at the end of the semester or school year, and later student progress was not reported. Studies that faded the intervention reported maintenance of treatment gains. However, little is known about maintenance in studies without fading techniques. More systematic research is needed to assess the importance of fading or other maintenance strategies, and to answer questions regarding long-term effects and generalizability of home-based reinforcement procedures.

Social Validity

With few exceptions, the use of school–home notes has resulted in substantial improvements in students' classroom behavior. The results from several studies suggested that the procedure was more effective than interventions conducted entirely within the school setting (Ayllon, Garber, & Pisor, 1975). However, researchers and clinicians have become increasingly concerned with the validity of behavioral interventions from a social or societal perspective. Assessments of social validity have considered the importance of treatment goals and effects and the appropriateness of treatment procedures (Elliott, 1988; Wolf, 1978).

Relatively few researchers have assessed the social validity of school–home notes. Although limited, data support the social validity of the procedure. For example, Lahey et al. (1977) reported that parents' responses to a questionnaire administered 7 weeks after treatment began indicated that they viewed the intervention as successful. The parents also indicated that the intervention was important to their children's education and had resulted in improved parent–teacher communication. Although parent satisfaction has been reported anecdotally in several studies, systematic evaluations of teachers' and students' satisfaction with the treatment or outcome have not been conducted.

In a few studies, the acceptability of school–home notes was compared to that of other classroom management techniques. Witt et al. (1984) obtained evaluations of the acceptability of six classroom interventions from 180 teachers. The subjects were presented with written case descriptions of a behavior problem child and were asked to evaluate the acceptability of a single treatment, using a 20-item scale. The data indicated that home-based reinforcement was perceived as highly acceptable and received higher ratings than a token economy, time out, or ignoring. However, school–home notes were not rated as highly as praise or response cost.

Turco and Elliott (1986) used a similar methodology to evaluate children's acceptance of home-based versus school-based contingency management procedures. Fifth-, seventh-, and ninth-graders evaluated the acceptability of a single intervention as applied to a written case vignette of a student with a behavior problem. Overall, the students preferred home-based praise over home-based reprimands, public teacher praise, and public teacher reprimands.

Although few investigators have examined this issue, research examining the social validity of school–home notes has been supportive. Parents report being satisfied with the procedure, and both teachers and students seem to view home-based contingency management as a highly acceptable method for remediating classroom behavior problems.

Many unanswered questions remain regarding the social validity of school–home notes. For example, it is unknown how teachers' or students' ratings of acceptability are influenced by experience with the intervention. Perhaps students (particularly adolescents), for example, would view the procedure as less acceptable if they were required to obtain teacher evaluations publicly. There is also a lack of information about whether variations in subject characteristics, school–home note format, or parent/teacher training would influence consumer acceptance.

SUMMARY

School–home reinforcement programs have several advantages over traditional, classroom-based contingency management systems. The procedure promotes parent-teacher communication and collaborative problem solving. School–home notes make use of the wide range of incentives available in the home. Because teachers are typically responsible for only a component of the treatment program, use of teacher time is very efficient.

This literature review suggests that school–home note procedures employed across studies have varied substantially. For example, the evaluation criteria used by teachers and the type of feedback provided to parents have ranged from global to specific. Similarly, training of parents and teachers in the proper use of school–home notes has varied from minimal contact to comprehensive programs. The relationship between these variables and the effectiveness of the procedure is unclear, as all of the studies reviewed reported successful results. In addition, few studies systematically examined the influence of procedural variables on treatment efficacy. The importance of component analyses was demonstrated by Blechman, Taylor, and Schrader (1981), who found that more extensive parent training was related to favorable treatment outcome.

The social validity of school–home notes also has not been thoroughly assessed. The relatively few studies in which the social validity of this procedure was examined support its use; however, additional evaluations comparing the social validity of school–home notes to that of other behavior interventions are needed.

Research evaluating the use of school–home notes has often contained methodological limitations. For example, very few studies assessed the integrity with which the intervention was employed through the monitoring of parent and teacher behavior. In several cases, the studies lacked adequate measurement of the dependent and independent variables. Finally, follow-up data were not reported.

In summary, school–home notes have been quite effective in remediating children's school problems and should be considered in the intervention plans of school-based practitioners wanting to elicit the assistance of both parents and teachers. Several methodological and clinical issues, however, warrant continued refinement of the procedure.

3

Assessment of School and Home Functioning

BEHAVIORAL ASSESSMENT

Researchers and clinicians often disagree about definitions of behavioral assessment and about what techniques encompass the approach. Several key features distinguish behavioral assessment from more traditional perspectives, however. Table 3.1 summarizes some of the differences between traditional and behavioral assessment (Hartmann, Roper, & Bradford, 1979). As suggested in Table 3.1, behavioral assessment emphasizes specifying behavior excesses and deficits and the situations in which these problem behaviors occur. As such, behavioral assessment often includes direct observation of behavior in the natural environment. Behavioral assessment also is conducted at a relatively molecular level in comparison to trait-oriented approaches, and similarly eschews the high level of inference about what behavior means that is characteristic of psychodynamic assessment. For example, behavioral psychologists usually will not describe a child's academic problems as simply due to "hyperactivity" or "depression." They also refrain from making inferences about underlying biological and structural deficits that affect learning, such as referring to a child's neurological dysfunction (Shapiro & Lentz, 1986).

Behavioral Versus Traditional Assessment: An Illustrative Example

The greater utility of behavioral assessment as opposed to traditional approaches is illustrated by the ways in which the two schools of

TABLE 3.1. Differences Between Behavioral and Traditional Approaches to Assessment

	Behavioral	Traditional
I. Assumptions		
1. Conception of personality	Personality constructs mainly employed to summarize specific behavior patterns, if at all	Personality as a reflection of enduring underlying states or traits
2. Causes of behavior	Maintaining conditions sought in current environment	Intrapsychic or within the individual
II. Implications		
1. Role of behavior	Important as a sample of person's repertoire in specific situation	Behavior assumes importance only insofar as it indexes underlying causes
2. Role of history	Relatively unimportant, except, for example, to provide a retrospective baseline	Crucial in that present conditions seen as a product of the past
3. Consistency of behavior	Behavior thought to be specific to the situation	Behavior expected to be consistent across time and settings
III. Uses of data	To describe target behaviors and maintain conditions	To describe personality functioning and etiology
	To select the appropriate treatment	To diagnose or classify
	To evaluate and revise treatment	To make prognosis; to predict
IV. Other characteristics		
1. Level of inferences	Low	Medium to high
2. Comparisons	More emphasis on intra-individual or idiographic	More emphasis on inter-individual or nomothetic
3. Methods of assessment	More emphasis on direct methods (e.g., observations of behavior in natural environment)	More emphasis on indirect methods (e.g., interviews and self-report)
4. Timing of assessment	More ongoing; prior, during, and after treatment	Pre- and perhaps posttreatment, or strictly to diagnose

TABLE 3.1. (continued)

	Behavioral	Traditional
5. Scope of assessment	Specific measures and of more variables (e.g., of target behaviors in various situations, of side effects, context, strengths as well as deficiencies)	More global measures (e.g., of cure or improvement), but only of the individual

Note. From "Source Relationships between Behavioral and Traditional Assessment" by D. P. Hartmann, B. L. Roper, and D. C. Bradford, 1979, *Journal of Behavioral Assessment, 1*, 3–21. Copyright 1979 by Plenum Press. Reprinted by permission.

thought might address the commonly encountered question, "Is my child hyperactive?" A psychologist who emphasizes the use of normative, traditional methods of testing, such as paper-and-pencil measures of attention deficit-hyperactivity disorder (ADHD), may answer the question with a simple "yes" or "no" based on test data. On the surface, a simple answer may seem satisfactory. However, it is likely that parents' and teachers' questions about diagnosis are prompted by concerns about such behaviors as the child's disruptiveness, aggressiveness, failure to complete classwork, or noncompliance. Thus, traditional approaches may simply end the assessment with classification and fail to identify the actual problem behaviors upon which the diagnosis is based. This lack of problem specification makes the development of an individualized treatment program tailored to the problems of the child impossible.

In contrast, consultants who emphasize a behavioral approach conduct more idiographic assessments. They may address parents' and teachers' concerns about hyperactivity by assessing the specific problems that have prompted teachers' and parents' inquiries. Although a comprehensive assessment may include the administration of norm-based measures of ADHD, the emphasis is on identifying specific behavior deficits, the setting in which the problems occur, and other functional factors (e.g., reinforcement contingencies). Thus, the child is labeled only to the extent that classification has a direct bearing on treatment outcome. Classification is rarely viewed as a fully adequate end result.

Behavioral Assessment as a Problem-Solving Tool

A primary feature of behavioral assessment is that it is a hypothesis-testing process that leads directly to problem solving (Shapiro & Kratochwill, 1988). Identifying problem behaviors and the settings in which problems occur brings treatment goals into the forefront. For example, by specifying "talking without permission" as the problem behavior, as opposed to labeling the child as "excessively demanding of attention" or "insecure," the consultant has a much clearer idea of what behavior to change.

Behavioral psychologists typically view assessment as a component of problem solving that ends with the implementation and evaluation of solutions. Gutkin and Curtis (1982), for example, describe a seven-step problem-solving process applicable to academic problems and classroom situations. As briefly outlined by Witt, Elliott, Gresham, and Kramer (1988), the steps are as follows:

1. Define the problem in clear, observable terms.
2. Determine the factors that appear to prompt, reward, punish, or in some other way influence problem behavior.
3. Generate strategies for problem solving.
4. Evaluate solutions and determine the best one.
5. Specify responsibilities of individuals involved in applying the chosen solution.
6. Employ the chosen solution.
7. Evaluate solution effectiveness and repeat the process if needed.

These problem-solving steps illustrate the link between assessment and treatment and show assessment as a process that continues after treatment begins. The steps also emphasize accountability through evaluation of treatment programs.

Elliott and Piersel's (1982) assessment funnel further illustrates the link between assessment and treatment. The assessment funnel, which sequences various assessment methods according to specificity, is shown in Figure 3.1. The funnel begins with the use of assessment techniques that yield general information about a wide range of potential problem behaviors. Information obtained at this level is mainly useful for screening and determining the focus of the assessment. As the funnel narrows, more detailed information is obtained, and hypotheses about the etiology and maintenance of problem behavior are refined.

Although Elliott and Piersel (1982) initially applied the funnel to the assessment of reading skills, the model can easily be extended to evaluating many childhood problems in the school and home environments. The model is noteworthy in three major ways. First, it emphasizes the inductive, idiographic assessment approach characteristic of a behavioral perspective. Second, the funnel shows the use of multiple assessment techniques (rather than just one or two) in a

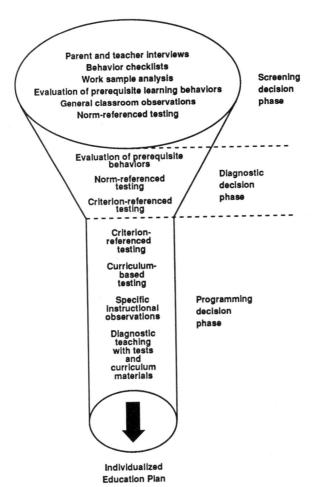

FIGURE 3.1. The assessment funnel. From "Direct Assessment of Reading Skills: An Approach Which Links Assessment to Intervention" by S. N. Elliott and W. C. Piersel, 1982, *School Psychology Review, 11,* pp. 257–280. Copyright 1982 by the National Association of School Psychologists. Reprinted by permission.

purpose-specific manner. Finally, the model ends with a proposed problem solution, which, in the case shown in Figure 3.1, is an individualized education plan.

Behavior Analysis

The major theoretical basis of behavioral assessment methods is found in the scientific approach called "behavior analysis." Although behavior analysis has been applied to the assessment and treatment of children's classroom problems for many years, clinicians and researchers often view the approach as one that is narrowly focused and only useful to understanding simple behavior problems. Behavior analysis often is seen as only concerned with observable behavior. Consultants working with children often view causes of behavior as either environmental or biological; thus, they dichotomize problems based on etiology. For example, some behavioral psychologists appear to ignore the effects of temperament or other biologically based factors on behavior. Likewise, more traditional psychologists often see behavior analysis as only relevant in situations where problems are very obviously maintained by reinforcing consequences and where other factors appear irrelevant. Both groups of consultants fail to appreciate the complex interplay among biological, behavioral (overt and covert), and environmental variables. I feel strongly that behavior analysis is a useful heuristic that can guide the assessment of psychological and biological variables relevant to the maintenance of children's behavior problems.

Figure 3.2 illustrates the model of behavior analysis used here, which takes into account the interplay among biological, behavioral, and environmental variables. This model was first presented in Kelley and Drabman (in press). Similar models are provided elsewhere (Bijou & Baer, 1978; Redd & Rusch, 1985).

As shown in Figure 3.2, the model suggests that any number of observable or unobservable events may serve as antecedents to behavior. For instance, antecedents precede target behavior and set the occasion for target behavior to occur. Antecedents to appropriate classroom performance may be a teacher's instructions or the child's reading of the directions.

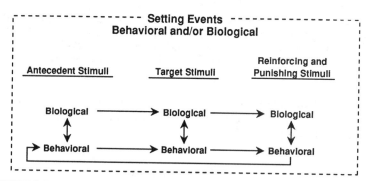

FIGURE 3.2. Model of behavior analysis. From "Psychological Contributions to Primary Pediatric Health Care" by M. L. Kelley and R. S. Drabman, unpublished manuscript.

Consequences are either (1) *reinforcing,* in which case the behavior they follow increases; or (2) *punishing,* in which case they result in decreases in target behavior. Like antecedents, consequences may be biological, behavioral, or environmental. For example, consider the situation in which a child fails to complete his or her classwork and instead talks to other children or doodles. The child's lack of work completion may be positively reinforced by enjoyable interactions with his or her peers and increased teacher attention in the form of prompts to begin working. The child's behavior is negatively reinforced because he or she avoids the aversive consequences associated with classwork. These consequences may include unobservable events (i.e., cognitions), such as the child's negative self-statements about his or her ability to complete the assignment. Assessment of the way in which behavior functions to produce reinforcing and punishing consequences is called a "functional analysis."

Setting events represent the context or setting in which behavior occurs. They are antecedent events that often do not *immediately* precede the behavior they influence (Bijou and Baer, 1978). For example, someone may have a very negative experience early in the day (e.g., a fight with the boss), and this event affects the person's behavior much later in the day (e.g., upon returning home from work). Setting events are antecedent events that influence behavior by altering the strength and characteristics of stimuli and responses. For example, a person who is hungry (setting event) will be more likely to eat (behavior) when offered a cookie (antecedent). Setting events may be physiological or temperament variables, such as a child's activity level, distractibility, or the presence of illness, fatigue, or hunger. For example, a child besieged by allergy symptoms may perform less competently across a wide variety of situations than when he or she is not symptomatic. Setting events may also be environmental circumstances, such as the location of the child's desk, the content of instructional material, or teacher presence versus absence in a classroom.

In addition, the behavior of others may serve as setting events. For example, numerous studies have shown that mothers' social interactions outside the home can affect their interactions with their children. On days when relatively isolated mothers experience frequent, friendly interactions with others, they behave more positively toward their children; their children, in turn, are more compliant and positive (Wahler, 1980). Many other family characteristics, such as maternal depression and marital conflict, influence children's behavior. Other interpersonal variables that may serve as setting events affecting children's classroom behavior include negative peer interactions, the presence of disruptive students in the classroom, and aversive parent–child interactions.

Several implications of the behavior-analytic model presented in Figure 3.2 should be emphasized here. First, the model can serve as an important way to integrate data from a variety of assessment sources. Second, the model is idiographic: The degree to which a given set of variables is functionally related to behavior may vary substantially across individuals or settings. Third, the model emphasizes the influence of setting events upon behavior, and thus can incorporate more molar, less immediate events into the behavioral formulation. Finally, the model acknowledges the complex interplay among biological, cognitive, and behavioral events without giving special status to any single event. For example, a child may be less likely to attend to stimuli across multiple situations, given his or her temperament and developmental status. This tendency may well be physiologically-based, but the physiological state is simply considered a setting event that influences the child's interactions with the environment.

In many respects, the behavior-analytic model put forth here is probably familiar to most readers. However, my colleagues and I have found the actual application of the model in clinical practice to be relatively infrequent. We consider the functional analysis of behavior to be an essential tool in effective clinical practice.

A Practical Application of the Behavior-Analytic Model

Recall the case presented in Chapter 1, in which Timothy often fails to complete his work and adhere to classroom rules. Both his parents and teacher have attempted to correct his behavior on numerous occasions. Apparently, Timothy completes his work on some occasions but not others, and therefore his teacher considers Timothy *able* to do the work. Frequently, behavior problems such as those exhibited by Timothy raise concerns as to whether the child suffers from "hyperactivity" or ADHD.

A functional analysis of Timothy's unsatisfactory work completion and classroom disruptiveness would probably suggest that his inappropriate behavior is maintained by numerous reinforcing consequences and is rarely punished. For example, a skilled observer sent into the classroom might note that the teacher and other students provide Timothy with a great deal of attention when he misbehaves. Inadequate reinforcement of appropriate behavior also may be seen. For instance, Timothy may fail to reinforce himself through positive self-talk for working diligently. Likewise, his teacher and parents may not praise him adequately or provide privileges in a contingent manner. Broadly based inventories or even an interview with the teacher might not detect some of these important features in Timothy's problems.

Timothy's greater distractibility and lack of attentiveness can be viewed as biologically based setting variables that influence his interactions with the environment. Altering these setting variables through the use of a pharmacological treatment, for example, may or may not produce substantial improvements in Timothy's behavior. It may be that Timothy will continue to misbehave or show only moderate improvements in his behavior with medication alone, in spite of his being more attentive and less active.

The example illustrates an idiographic assessment approach—one that incorporates biological, cognitive, and behavioral variables into the analysis. When certain biological variables are viewed as setting events that affect subsequent interactions, the effects of such factors as temperament, intellectual functioning, illness, and the like are acknowledged without (1) giving these events a special status; (2) adopting the dualistic mind—body approach to assessment that is characteristic of the medical model; or (3) taking an "either—or" approach, whereby one factor is held responsible for the observed problem.

ADDITIONAL ASSESSMENT CONSIDERATIONS

Thus far, I have emphasized the use of evaluation techniques that lead directly to treatment. The discussion has been broadly based and intended to provide a general framework for determining when, where, and how to assess children's academic performance and classroom behavior. In order to conduct a comprehensive, accurate assessment of the factors maintaining a specific child's behavior problems, a number of other assessment issues must be addressed. This section of the chapter highlights some of the most important areas to include in a comprehensive school and home assessment. For the reader's convenience, I have included an interview guide for use with parents in Appendix 3.1. Addressing these issues will give the consultant a much better idea about specific ways of including parents and teachers in the behavior change process.

Direct Assessment of Academic Skills

To an extent, a consultant's decision to include a school–home note system in a child's treatment program will depend on the degree to which the child's behavior can be improved through increased parental reinforcement. In order to make this determination, the consultant must ascertain whether the child can perform necessary academic skills. That is, the consultant must determine the degree to which the child's problems are due to performance deficits versus academic skill deficits. For example, a child's failing mathematics grade may be due to an inability to multiply two-digit numbers or to an unwillingness to use skills he or she possesses. When the child's behavior problems are largely due to skill deficits, school–home notes may be used as a secondary intervention designed to promote academic skill acquisition. However, children's academic problems are rarely due to skill deficits only. Reinforcement such as that required in behavioral shaping frequently accelerates skill acquisition and performance. This process can be enhanced through increased parent involvement in the program.

A relatively recent trend in the school psychology literature is a move away from traditional techniques for assessing academic skills and toward the use of more behavioral, direct assessment approaches. According to Shapiro and Lentz (1986), direct assessment of academic skills must do the following:

> Involve direct observation of the academic behavior, utilize work samples produced in the natural environment, provide behavioral targets for intervention, be based on the curriculum in which the individual is having problems, be capable of frequent repetition, be based on empirical research and include an assessment of environmental variables. (p. 91)

Shapiro and Lentz (1986), like numerous other authors who advocate direct assessment of academic skills, recommend the use of curriculum-based testing and frequent monitoring of student skill acquisition throughout the treatment process (e.g., Fuchs & Fuchs, 1986; Shapiro, 1988; Witt & Bartlett, 1982). These authors state that data obtained from norm-referenced tests, such as measures of intelligence and achievement, are inadequate for conducting a functional analysis of academic skill deficits. Three sources of information materials for conducting curriculum-based assessment are recommended: (1) criterion-referenced or mastery tests that accompany texts; (2) assessment probes derived directly from the curriculum; and (3) published criterion-referenced tests such as the KeyMath Diagnostic Test. (The reader is directed to Shapiro & Lentz, 1986, for a thorough discussion of the mechanics of conducting curriculum-based assessment.)

Direct assessment of academic skills also requires a careful analysis of the environmental events associated with behavior. For example, the amount of classroom time children spend engaged in academic activities such as working mathematics problems has a direct bearing on achievement and should be evaluated when academic problem areas are reported. Careful assessment of antecedents to academic responses, such as the quality and content of instruction, is also important (Shapiro & Lentz, 1986). With regard to consequences, the consultant should evaluate frequency of teacher feedback and reinforcement and the degree to which the child is reinforced for engaging in behavior incompatible with academic productivity. Additional examples of areas to assess are shown in the teacher interview guide (Shapiro & Lentz, 1986) presented in Table 3.2.

Direct assessment of academic skills focuses on determining the child's current skill level and the environmental variables associated with academic performance such as amount of instruction. The emphasis, quite naturally, is on the classroom environment, the child as a student, and academic productivity. A host of additional teacher, family, and student variables may affect children's classroom performance, however. Because treatment may include a variety of behaviors in addition to academic productivity, the next three sections discuss some of these other variables.

Teacher Variables

In addition to curriculum and method of instruction, teachers may affect children's classroom performance in many ways. Teachers often remark that they are only human, with the implication being that they are not impervious to excessive job demands and unappreciative, uncooperative parents and students (and consultants!).

Teachers' degree of cooperativeness with consultants also depends on a variety of organizational factors. These factors include administrative support and attitudes of school personnel toward teacher involvement in behavior modification programs (Gutkin, Clark, & Achenbaum, 1985). Although teacher variables are not easy to assess, consultants must be sensitive to them when planning and employing classroom interventions.

Hawryluk and Smallwood (1986) identify four aspects of teacher functioning that should be included in school-based assessments: knowledge, skills, cognition, and affect. For example, the consultant should consider the effects of administrative policies and availability of system resources in the functional analysis. Teacher variables can

TABLE 3.2. Teacher Interview for Academic Assessment

Academic Subject:_____

<u>Assessing Materials and Progress Monitoring</u>

    Curriculum materials used:_____

    Teaching procedures:_____

    Time allotted/day:_____

    Year-end goals:_____

    Describe monitoring procedure:_____

    How is placement determined?:_____

    What is present placement?:_____

    How is mastery assessed?:_____

<u>Contingencies for Academic Performance</u>

    Typical daily assignment:_____

    Contingency accuracy:_____

    Contingency for completion:_____

    Type of feedback:_____

<u>Expected Performance Levels</u>

    Grade level of present placement:_____
    Grade level expected by teacher
      at present time:_____

    Teacher satisfaction with progress:_____

<u>Other Data</u>

    Daily scores (if available) for
      past two weeks:_____

    Standardized test results:_____
    How are changes made in
      academic program?:_____

Note. From "Behavioral Assessment of Academic Skills" by E. S. Shapiro and F. E. Lentz, 1986, in T. R. Kratochwill (Ed.), *Advances in school psychology* (Vol. 5, pp. 87–139). Hillsdale, NJ: Erlbaum. Copyright 1986 by Lawrence Erlbaum Associates. Reprinted by permission.

have a very direct bearing on the type of treatment one chooses to solve a child's classroom problem. The discussion below highlights some of the factors discussed by Hawryluk and Smallwood (1986).

The consultant must determine the extent to which the teacher is knowledgeable about the target student, relevant educational programs, and school and community resources. For example, is the teacher aware of the student's academic strengths and weaknesses and of relevant family and cultural characteristics? Is the teacher knowledgeable about curriculum materials, classroom management techniques, and effective teaching strategies? On one occasion, I was asked to treat a first-grade boy who failed to complete his classwork in a timely manner. Teacher interviews and classroom observations revealed that the teacher required students to spend most of the morning working independently on assignments listed on the chalkboard. The students received very little feedback during this time; instead, the teacher conducted reading groups or graded papers. The target child was only one of several students who were failing to work productively during this morning work period. The teacher believed that students should be able to complete the work without close supervision or praise for productive, appropriate behavior. Interviews with the teacher made it clear that she lacked sufficient knowledge about child development and classroom instruction to be an effective teacher.

Even when teachers possess adequate knowledge, they may lack adequate skill for effective teaching, classroom management, and implementing a behavioral program. For example, the consultant should assess whether the teacher is sufficiently organized to teach effectively while simultaneously implementing a behavioral program. The teacher must be interpersonally competent in such areas as self-control and problem-solving, and must be able to elicit parent and student cooperation. For example, a teacher may agree to evaluate a student's behavior on a daily basis, yet may fail to carry through with the commitment consistently and accurately. In cases where my colleagues and I encountered this problem, we erroneously presumed that the teacher was adequately organized and committed to a school–home note system. Had we more carefully assessed the teacher's organizational and problem-solving skills, implementation problems (e.g., increased parental irritation with the teacher) could have been avoided.

Less overt variables also may influence teacher interest and cooperation. As Hawryluk and Smallwood (1986) suggest, it is important to assess teachers' beliefs and expectations about students, their teaching responsibilities, and expectations for client assessment and treatment. Unfounded, biased beliefs may prevent teachers from using their knowledge and skills. For example, a teacher may prematurely and erroneously conclude that a child lacks skills for adequate classroom functioning, and may believe that special education is the only viable treatment alternative. In this case, treatment efforts, such as employing a school–home note system, may be ineffective solely because of a lack of teacher cooperation.

Inappropriate teacher expectations and irrational beliefs about the causes of problem behavior were also seen in the example above in which the teacher required lengthy periods of independent seatwork from first-graders. In this example, the teacher inaccurately concluded that the target child's lack of productivity was due to lax disciplining by the parents. She was resistant to changing her behavior or classroom routine. The only solution she was willing to accept was increased punishment by the parents, the school principal, or herself.

Like that of any employee, teachers' job performance and motivation may be affected by personal factors other than those immediately present in the problem situation. Low morale may decrease teachers' performance in general and cooperation with the consultation process in particular. Personal problems such as depression, marital difficulties, illness, or other sources of stress may adversely affect instruction, classroom management, and teachers' willingness to implement behavioral interventions. Teachers may not react positively if a consultant inquires directly about personal problems. On the other hand, if a teacher gives off signals of being under stress, a few sympathetic remarks about the trials of the teaching profession may help establish rapport leading to a productive working relationship. In any case, the consultant should remain cognizant of the effects of stress and personal problems on teachers' performance, and should attempt to create a supportive environment so that these problems may be sensitively discussed if they should arise.

Parent and Family Variables

When a child's academic performance, classroom behavior, or positive peer interactions decline, a teacher often asks, "How are things at home?" If the teacher is aware of changes or turmoil in the child's environment, such as marital conflict or the death of a grandparent, the teacher *and* parents very commonly attribute declines in performance to these negative events. Negative events do influence children's ability to function in the classroom, just as they do adults' job performance. Consequently, it is important to assess the extent to which family variables are contributing to classroom failure and to determine whether they will interfere with treatment that does not focus directly on family problems.

Demographic Variables

The consultant should be sensitive to the diverse demographic and cultural variables that may affect the student's performance and parents' responsivity to assessment and treatment. For example, it is important to determine the family's income status and housing situation; poverty is associated with a number of factors that directly affect academic success. The child may live in a crowded environment where there is little opportunity for completing schoolwork in a quiet setting. The child may live in a single-parent home where the parent (typically the mother) has little time to spend with him or her because of working two jobs and caring for other children.

It is also important to determine the parents' educational background and academic skills. For example, a parent's reading ability may affect the ways in which the consultant involves parents in treatment; parents who do not read may not be able to assist with homework completion. In assessing demographic variables, the consultant should inquire about other adults who assist with child care, as well as other family resources. Sometimes children receive a good deal of attention from neighbors or relatives, and these individuals may be available to assist with treatment.

The literature indicates that poverty, single-parent status, and a limited educational background are associated with poor treatment outcome; parents with these characteristics often do not follow through with treatment recommendations. Although these parents may be less likely to implement treatment recommendations than middle-class parents, I strongly believe that premature assumptions should not be made about their ability and interest in promoting their children's academic progress. I take the stance that poorly educated parents are not necessarily poor candidates for assisting with treatment. My colleagues and I have been involved in numerous cases in which the mothers' limited education and impoverishment did not impede their ability to implement a school–home note system. These mothers showed very good problem-solving skills, as evidenced by having overcome many obstacles. For example, one mother with several children in a small home arranged for her son to complete his schoolwork at the home of a relative.

Parental Distress and Psychopathology

A number of factors related to parental adjustment are associated with ineffective parenting and poor treatment prognosis. These factors include maternal depression, social isolation, and high levels of stress, all of which should be assessed prior to making treatment recommendations. When depressed, a mother may view her child more negatively. Depressed mothers also interact more negatively with their children and are less likely to use recommended parenting techniques. Other factors correlated with mothers' negative perceptions of their children and poor parenting are marital conflict and a lack of spouse support (Forehand, Brody & Smith, 1986; Furey & Forehand, 1984; Kelley, Embry, & Baer, 1979).

In our own research as well as that of others, mothers who report experiencing a large number of negative events or who lack adequate social support are less likely to behave positively toward their children or to benefit from parent training (Dumas & Wahler, 1985; Kelley & Carper, 1988; Wahler, 1980). This relationship between negative events and negative behavior appears to occur on a daily basis within a particular family and may affect whether a mother will use positive child management techniques (Dumas & Wahler, 1983; Wahler, 1980; Wahler & Afton, 1980).

Although these variables often interfere with treatment success and should be considered in treatment planning, it is unfair to assume that distressed mothers will be unable to follow through with treatment recommendations. In fact, a number of mothers whom we counseled reported feeling less distressed and depressed as a result of using our suggestions for more effectively interacting with their children. Also, as their children's behavior improved, the mothers reported seeing themselves as more competent and consequently became less depressed. (The reader is directed to Forehand, 1987, for a more comprehensive discussion of the effects of parent maladjustment on children's behavior.)

Parental Expectations

As with teachers, it is important to determine parents' expectations of their child and their perceived role in promoting academic success. For example, does a parent view the school as primarily responsible for solving the child's academic problems? Particularly in situations where contact with families is initiated by the school, parents may not view a school–home note system or any other parenting procedure as an important, appropriate way of remediating children's academic difficulties. In such instances, my colleagues and I attempt to reach a consensus among the interested parties as to the school's versus the parents' role in increasing children's classroom functioning.

For a variety of reasons, parents sometimes believe they are incapable of solving their children's problems, and therefore resist involvement in treatment. They may feel that they have already tried every viable approach without success. Parents may also believe that there is something inherently wrong with their children (e.g., learning disabilities, hyperactivity) or the teachers (e.g., "She hates my child") that prevents them from helping to solve their children's academic problems. They may believe that the only solution is medication, some other medical procedure, or a "special" program. Parents also may view rewarding children's appropriate behavior as unnecessary, because they feel that children should not be bribed or given special attention for performing expected tasks.

Dealing with parents who express negative beliefs about treatment can be very frustrating. It is our experience that confronting these parents directly about their beliefs simply adds fuel to their resistance. Instead, we tend to empathize with how frustrating the situation has been for them; to address their reservations in a straightforward, sincere manner; and to sensitively point out ways in which they might view themselves and their children more constructively.

Parenting Knowledge and Skills

It is important to assess parents' ability to discipline their children in an effective, consistent manner. For example, the consultant should ask whether noncompliance is generally a problem and whether instructions must be repeated numerous times before they are obeyed. The parents should be asked about the methods they normally use to punish and reward behavior, as well as about the consistency with which they use the techniques. By evaluating parenting effectiveness, the consultant is able to plan the extent to which skills training will be a necessary component of treatment.

It is helpful to assess whether parents have established routines, such as for bedtime and homework. If structured routines do not exist, it may be difficult to implement a school–home note system, because the procedure requires consistency and structure.

My colleagues and I recommend evaluating the frequency and quality of parent–child interactions in child-directed (e.g., play) situations as well. For example, the consultant should attempt to determine whether parents are overbearing or overprotective during their children's unstructured activities. Also, how often do the family members engage in enjoyable activities and interact positively with one another? Do the parents take an active interest in discussing their children's daily activities without criticizing the children or intrusively solving their problems for them?

It may be that parent–child interactions are generally negative and that schoolwork is just another area where the parents attempt to use punitive procedures to prompt appropriate behavior. In these cases, it may be necessary to address general parenting deficits prior to beginning a school–home note system.

Spouse inconsistency and a lack of spouse involvement in child rearing can also contribute to children's oppositional behavior and lack of adaptive functioning. For this reason, it is important to evaluate the degree to which the mother and father support each other's disciplining attempts, are equally effective and positive, and share similar expectations for their children. For example, does one parent generally discipline the child? Does the child manipulate the parents in order to get his or her way?

When children are having academic problems, homework often becomes a primary source of marital conflict. In these cases, the child is uncooperative and dawdles when expected to work on homework. Sometimes homework ends up taking a great deal of one parent's time, which is resented by the spouse. Other times, the parents disagree about how much help and supervision should be provided during homework, or how to handle behavior problems such as crying, dawdling, and complaining.

A frequently occurring problem is that fathers are unwilling to participate in treatment or to implement recommended parenting procedures. Although this does not necessarily preclude mothers from administering a behavioral program, uninvolved fathers can impede their spouses' participation by criticizing or sabotaging recommended treatments. In order to facilitate parent cooperation, the consultant should attempt to interview both parents during all phases of assessment and treatment, and should work to obtain fathers' cooperation and involvement.

Other Family Variables

A variety of less common problems can also affect children's academic performance and the parents' ability to participate effectively in treatment. Almost any significant life event or change in a child's routine may affect his or her classroom behavior. These problems include substance abuse, divorce or remarriage, and recent death or illness of a relative. It is good practice to inquire about changes within the family, particularly if the child's decline in academic performance is recent and sudden.

Parents are sometimes defensive when the consultant asks about family problems. They may fail to recognize the relevance of their behavior to their children's academic functioning. I usually address this problem by explaining to parents that a variety of circumstances may affect children's behavior and that it is very helpful to know about *any* situation affecting the family or the child. I address the issues of marital conflict, maternal depression, parental expectations, and other family variables in a straightforward, assertive manner.

Parents sometimes avoid revealing relevant information during initial sessions, in spite of the consultant's efforts to establish rapport through the use of direct yet sensitive questioning. For example, on several occasions I discovered long after treatment was initiated that a parent had a serious substance abuse problem. In these cases, the nonabusing parent actively participated in treatment and made excuses for the lack of direct involvement of the other parent (e.g., "He has to work"). In one case when the father was hospitalized for drug abuse, I asked the mother why she had not told us about the problem. She stated that she believed it probably accounted for only about 20% of the child's problems and therefore was not terribly relevant. In actuality, the mother attempted to *make up* for her husband's behavior through her enthusiastic involvement in a school–home note program. Initially, she did not wish to address the substance abuse problem in a direct manner and hoped that she could change her son's behavior without focusing on the larger context.

Sometimes children's classroom behavior problems can be improved without addressing more serious family problems. However, many times, as in the case noted above, a tightly focused approach is ineffective. Because parents are sometimes reluctant to disclose problems during initial sessions, we repeat our inquiry about family functioning when treatment is ineffective or the functional analysis appears incomplete.

Child Variables

Children bring to their environments unique characteristics that may consistently affect their behavior across many situations. For example, a child's tendency to be distractible or shy may be evidenced across a wide range of situations. As stated earlier in this chapter, these global characteristics may be viewed as setting variables that affect the child's later interactions. Numerous characteristics may serve as setting events, including depression, ADHD, substance abuse, and anxiety. Obviously, this chapter cannot adequately review the assessment of these disorders. Instead, the assessment of ADHD and depression— two frequently encountered problems—are briefly described.

In interviewing parents and teachers, we recommend evaluating the severity, chronicity, and cross-situationality of children's behavior problems. If the child's behavior is problematic across a wide variety of situations, extremely severe in some situations, relatively stable across time, and/or seemingly resistant to treatment efforts, behavioral interventions focusing strictly on academic and classroom behavior problems are likely to be only moderately effective. In these situations, a multimodal treatment approach involving parents, teachers, and the child is probably necessary.

Attention Deficit–Hyperactivity Disorder

With regard to ADHD, we suggest that the consultant maintain an idiographic assessment focus that leads to an individualized treatment plan. In addition to directly assessing the child's academic skills, it is recommended that the assessment procedure include (1) comprehensive parent, teacher, and child interviews aimed at generating a specific problem list and relevant functional variables; (2) norm-referenced assessment of ADHD using parents and teachers as informants; (3) direct observations in the classroom and playground in order to determine the degree to which the child's behavior deviates from the norm, and to gather information on problem behavior and the contingencies maintaining the behavior; and (4) collection of observational data on parent–child interactions in the home setting, when it is possible and relevant.

In assessing ADHD, the issue should not be one of simply determining whether to medicate the child, but rather one of conducting an individualized assessment and treatment. This is not to imply, however, that the use of medication necessarily excludes a behavioral perspective, or vice versa. In dealing with children who are very difficult to manage because of their extreme distractibility, impulsivity, and disruptive behavior, a treatment combining medication and behavior management may result in optimal effects (Pelham, 1984). For example, a combined behavioral–pharmacological treatment approach may result in behavior that more closely approximates the norm than that produced by either treatment alone. In addition, we have found that individualized school–home notes are useful in assessing behavior before and during treatment. They can be used as a record form for evaluating the effects of various interventions, such as a contingency management program and medication. (For a more comprehensive discussion of the assessment and treatment of ADHD see Barkley, 1988; Gadow, 1988; and Schaughency, Walker, & Lahey, 1988. See also Chapter 5, this volume.)

Depression

Depression in children can result in markedly diminished functioning, including an inability to cope with the academic and social demands of school. Although depression is a much more common cause of poor school performance in adolescents than in children, the literature suggests that significant levels of depressive symptomatology can be evidenced in young elementary school children. Thus, depression should not be overlooked as a possible reason for declining school performance, particularly when behavior changes occur over a relatively short period of time in a child with a history of satisfactory academic performance. In screening for problems of depression or other, less overt problems (e.g., negative self-evaluation, significant anxiety problems), the consultant should rely extensively on the interview with the child as a source of data. In general, the usefulness of information provided by children increases with age, and self-report should be an integral part of the assessment process with a teenager.

ASSESSMENT PROCEDURES

Thus far, I have described and recommended a behavioral assessment approach for evaluating children's classroom problems and have discussed specific variables that should be included in the functional analysis. This section of the chapter outlines specific assessment methods that aid problem-solving, with emphasis on behavioral rather than traditional assessment devices. The methods discussed are behavioral interview techniques and formats, paper-and-pencil instruments, and direct observation. Additional methods are briefly mentioned. Specific measures for assessing intellectual functioning and academic achievement are not emphasized. The discussion is intended to be illustrative rather than exhaustive.

Behavioral Interviews

Interviews have long been an important method used by school psychologists to gather information about children's classroom functioning (Gresham, 1984). However, consultative interviews often are unstructured and vague. Such interviews do not yield specific information about children's behavior (Gresham & Davis, 1988). In contrast, a behavioral interview emphasizes collecting data pertinent to the functional analysis and avoids vague discussions about children's personality. The interview is an essential assessment tool used to gather information that will lead directly to problem-solving, as well as to the planning and evaluation of treatment programs.

The behavioral interview format most often used to assess school problems is that of Bergan and his colleagues (Bergan, 1977; Bergan & Tombari, 1975). These authors propose a consultation format that encompasses the problem-solving model presented earlier. Behavioral consultation focuses on identifying specific problem behaviors and settings as well as on generating problem solutions (Feld, Bergan, & Stone, 1987). Bergan's behavioral consultation approach consists of four stages: (1) problem identification, (2) problem analysis, (3) plan implementation, and (4) problem evaluation. It is assumed that these steps will be accomplished in three interviews, each of which has a distinct purpose (Gresham & Davis, 1988). Although Bergan's interview format is limited in certain ways (e.g., the model does not emphasize assessment of setting events and focuses narrowly on the assessment of the school environment), it is well supported by research and serves as an excellent problem-solving guide. As such, the guidelines for conducting the three interviews are presented here as a heuristic rather than as a formula to follow rigidly.

Problem Identification Interview

In many respects, the first interview is the most important, because it sets the stage for all future consultation (Gresham & Davis, 1988). Adequate problem identification is directly related to successful treatment (Bergan & Tombari, 1975). Tables 3.3 and 3.4 summarize the components of problem identification that lead to accomplishing goals (Gresham & Davis, 1988).

As indicated in Table 3.3, the overall purpose of this interview is to identify specific problem behaviors and maintaining events. To accomplish this goal, it is necessary to ask questions that elicit information about specific and observable behavior, rather than to discuss problems using vague and inferential language. For example, the consultant might ask, "What does Timothy do that makes you think he is hyperactive?" or "In what situations does Timothy talk without permission?"

In addition to conducting a functional analysis of the child's behavior deficits and excesses, the consultation team should agree on methods of collecting data. Often, data-recording sheets are set up so that they may be used as school–home notes after baseline data collection. For example, we have used the note shown in Figure 1.1 (see Chapter 1) to collect baseline data. When the school–home note is

TABLE 3.3. Components of Problem Identification

I. *Explain purpose of consultation.*
   A. Provide overview and rationale.
   B. Focus upon client behavior.

II. *Identify and select target behaviors.*
   A. Define behavior in specific operational terms.
   B. Identify amount of discrepancy between behavior and goal.
   C. Prioritize behaviors to target.

III. *Identify frequency, duration, and intensity of behavior.*
   A. Obtain specific, objective information.
   B. Compare behavior rates with other students' behavior.
   C. Provide feedback on realistic expectations.

IV. *Identify environmental variables.*
   A. Specify antecedents and consequences.
   B. Specify setting events.

V. *Identify goals.*
   A. Determine expectations for change.
   B. Set specific criteria for reaching goals.
   C. Set time lines.

VI. *Identify client's strengths.*
   A. Remind consultee of client's assets.
   B. Detect negative biases.

VII. *Determine reinforcers.*
   A. Identify reinforcers available to consultee.
   B. Identify reinforcers meaningful to child.

VIII. *Identify methods of data collection.*
   A. Specify how and when to record.
   B. Specify what to record.

IX. *Identify consultee effectiveness.*

X. *Summarize accomplishments of meeting.*

XI. *Schedule a follow-up meeting.*

Note. Adapted from "Behavioral Interviews with Teachers and Parents" by F. M. Gresham and C. J. Davis, 1988, in E. S. Shapiro and T. R. Kratochwill (Eds.), *Behavioral Assessment in Schools: Conceptual Foundations and Practical Applications* (pp. 455–493). New York: Guilford Press. Copyright 1988 by The Guilford Press. Adapted by permission. Also adapted from "Assessment in Behavioral Consultation: The Initial Interview" by J. C. Witt and S. N. Elliott, 1983, *School Psychology Review, 12,* 42–49. Copyright 1983 by the National Association of School Psychologists. Adapted by permission.

TABLE 3.4. Effective Interviewing Behaviors

1. Ask *direct, specific questions* about the problem.

    Examples: "What does Charles do when he disturbs the class?"
    "Describe Johnny's hyperactive behavior."

2. Ask questions about *antecedents and consequences.*

    Examples: "What happens before Egbert begins to hit other children?"
    "What do you do after Egbert hits a student?"

3. Ask questions about *situational factors.*

    Examples: "During which subjects do you notice Johnny is most in-attentive?"
    "Who is Egbert with when he begins hitting other children?"

4. Ask questions about the *frequency and duration.*

    Examples: "How many times each day does Charles race around the room?"
    "How long will Susan stay on-task before beginning talking?"

5. Ask questions about *goals.*

    Example: "How much of a reduction in off-task behavior would you like to see?"

6. Ask questions regarding the *student's strengths.*

    Examples: "What are some things that Mary does do well?"
    "What are some of Egbert's assets?"

7. Ask questions about *teaching procedures.*

    Examples: "How long are Charles and the other students required to do seatwork?"
    "What is the order of subjects presented?"

8. Ask questions about *data collection.*

    Examples: "How would it be most convenient for you to keep a record of Charles's out-of-seat behavior?"
    "For what time periods and how long will you record the number of times Charles gets out of his chair?"

9. *Summarize* obtained information.

    Examples: "Let's see, the main problem is that Charles gets out of his seat and runs around the room during independent work assignments about four times each day. Is that right?"
    "You will record for 1 week the number of times Egbert hits other students in the morning before school and at noon."

Note. Adapted from "Behavioral Interviews with Teachers and Parents" by F. M. Gresham and C. J. Davis, 1988, in E. S. Shapiro and T. R. Kratochwill (Eds.), *Behavioral Assessment in Schools: Conceptual Foundations and Practical Applications* (pp. 455–493). New York: Guilford Press. Copyright 1988 by The Guilford Press. Adapted by permission.

adapted for data collection, parents, teachers, and students become familiar with the target behaviors and student performance. When the note is brought home for the parents to review prior to treatment, the consultant can assess the likelihood that the consultees will employ the procedure consistently. For example, if parents and teachers agreed that the note would be completed and brought home for an entire week, but it was sent home only twice, the consultant knows to address the problem of treatment integrity in subsequent interviews.

Problem Analysis Interview

The second interview has four objectives that lead directly from those accomplished during the problem identification phase. This interview usually occurs after the collection of baseline data. The overall purpose of the problem analysis interview is to refine the definitions of the problem and to develop and begin implementing a remediation plan. According to Gresham and Davis (1988), the specific goals of the problem analysis interview are these:

1. Validate the existence of a problem by evaluating baseline data and comparing the child's behavior to that of other children.
2. Very thoroughly analyze the conditions in which problem behavior occurs.
3. Design an intervention for improving behavior and detail precisely how the plan will be implemented.
4. Arrange for a subsequent meeting to evaluate treatment progress and further refine treatment procedures.

Gresham and Davis (1988) point out that teachers and parents are more likely to implement a treatment with integrity if they have participated in treatment selection. For example, the results of a study by Bergan (1977) showed that teachers were more likely to discuss resources for implementing a plan when the consultant elicited teachers' opinions about problem solutions.

Problem Evaluation Interview

The problem evaluation interview has four specific objectives (Gresham & Davis, 1988):

1. Determine whether the consultation goals have been achieved. If the goals have not been attained, then the consultant must reconsider his or her functional analysis of the problem and determine whether the intervention has been implemented appropriately.

2. Systematically evaluate intervention effectiveness by comparing baseline to treatment data. For example, what percentage of math problems did the child complete before and after treatment, and is this change adequate compared to other children's productivity rates?

3. Determine specific plans for continued treatment efforts. The consultation team may decide to continue, modify, or terminate treatment. Accomplishing this objective requires problem solving and direct communication among all parties involved.

4. Schedule additional sessions as needed.

The overall purpose of the interview is to evaluate how well the treatment is working. The interview usually takes place after treatment has been given sufficient time to begin working (approximately 1–2 weeks). A treatment often fails because it has not been used for an adequate period of time. We have found that some consultants and consultees withdraw an intervention that is not working, instead of refining it to increase treatment efficacy. This is unfortunate, because potentially effective treatments are rejected prematurely rather than modified to solve the problem. Parents and teachers should be told that treatments may not be immediately effective and often must be revised before they work. They should be encouraged to continue an intervention for a reasonable period of time (Gresham & Davis, 1988). Thus, in actuality, the problem evaluation phase of consultation may consist of several sessions in which unforeseen problems are addressed and interventions are revised or refined. It is rare for a single evaluation session to suffice, and it is shortsighted not to conduct additional sessions to follow up treatment successes.

Additional Interview Considerations

A variety of assessment issues must be considered during the interviews with parents and teachers. Many issues, such as those noted earlier in this chapter, require significant departures from the Bergan (1977) consultation model. For example, the strict application of Bergan's model for consultation is probably insufficient for interviewing a depressed mother whose husband is not supportive and sabotages her attempts to remediate their children's academic problems. However, viewing the consultation objectives as goals that must be eventually accomplished in order to remediate children's behavior problems can bring a necessary focus to the assessment and treatment process. I view the interviewer's task as one superimposed on the Bergan (1977) model.

A variety of additional issues must be considered when planning and conducting interviews with teachers, parents, and students. For example, the consultant must be skilled at promoting children's cooperation with school–home notes and at facilitating positive communication and negotiation between parents and teachers. The interviewer must have clear guidelines for determining when school versus home behavior problems are to be dealt with concurrently or sequentially. The consultant must be able to offer advice quickly and effectively about dealing with any number of home and school problems that may affect children's school performance. These include dealing with homework and bedtime problems and answering parents' questions about child development. (For a more detailed discussion of the behavioral consultation model and interviewing parents and teachers, see Feld et al., 1987; Gresham, 1984; and Gresham & Davis, 1988.)

Paper-and-Pencil Instruments

The use of psychometrically sound questionnaires has several advantages over less formal procedures. Checklists can be an efficient way to screen for family and child problems outside of the major assessment focus and to compare parents' and teachers' perceptions of a child's behavior to that of other children. By standardizing *what* questions are asked and *how,* questionnaires help insure that the information obtained from respondents is less variable and more accurate (Edelbrock, 1988). It is important to note that although scores derived from questionnaires are useful for screening and treatment evaluation, they are *not* diagnostic indices or adequately specific for inclusion in a functional analysis.

I recommend the use of several questionnaires for screening children with classroom behavior problems. Many of the instruments I have found useful for screening as well as for obtaining normative information are listed in Table 3.5. In almost all instances, I recommend that prior to treatment, parents and teachers complete some form of the Child Behavior Checklist (CBCL; Achenbach & Edelbrock, 1983, 1986, 1987) or the Eyberg Child Behavior Inventory (ECBI; Eyberg & Robinson, 1983; Robinson, Eyberg, & Ross, 1980). The CBCL assesses general psychopathology and has separate norms for boys and girls at different ages. Although the teacher and parent versions of the CBCL yield somewhat different factors, the information obtained from the two sources can be meaningfully compared. The authors have also developed a self-report version of the CBCL for youths aged 11–16. I suggest that this measure be included when target students are in the appropriate age range.

TABLE 3.5. Paper-and-Pencil Instruments Commonly Used in the Assessment of Child and Family Behavior Problems

Inventory	References	Content
Child self-report		
Child Behavior Checklist (CBCL) Youth Self-Report	Achenbach & Edelbrock (1983, 1987)	120-item measure of a wide range of behavior problems in adolescents aged 11–18
Children's Depression Inventory (CDI)	Kovacs (1983); Kovacs & Beck (1977)	27-item measure of children's depression
Reynolds Adolescent Depression Scale	Reynolds & Coats (1985)	30-item measure of depression in adolescents aged 12–17
Beck Depression Inventory (BDI)	Beck, Ward, Mendelson, Mock, & Erbaugh (1961)	21-item measure of depression for adolescents and adults
Revised Children's Manifest Anxiety Scale	Reynolds & Richmond (1978)	37-item general measure of anxiety for children and adolescents aged 6–17
Conflict Behavior Questionnaire	Prinz, Foster, Kent, & O'Leary (1979)	20-item forced-choice measure of parent–adolescent communication and conflict behavior.
Issues Checklist	Enyart (1984); Prinz et al. (1979); Enyart (1984)	44-item measure of the frequency and anger intensity of specific parent–adolescent conflict areas
Multidimensional Self-Concept Scale	Gresham, Elliott, & Evans (in press)	50-item measure of academic, social, and physical self-efficacy, as well as outcome expectations and general self-concept
Piers-Harris Children's Self-Concept Scale	Piers & Harris (1964)	80-item measure of self-concept for children and adolescents in the 4th through 12th grades
Social Skills Rating System	Gresham & Elliott (in press)	Self-report of social skills for children and adolescents in 3rd through 12th grades. Includes the following factors: Cooperation, Assertion, Empathy, and Self-Control
Adolescent Activity Checklist	Carey, Kelley, Buss, & Scott (1986)	100-item measure of pleasant and unpleasant events experienced by adolescents in 7th through 12th grades

TABLE 3.5. *(continued)*

Parent report		
CBCL Parent Report	Achenbach (1984); Achenbach & Edelbrock (1983)	120-item checklist of a wide variety of behavior problems in children and adolescents aged 2–16
Behavior Problem Checklist	Quay & Peterson (1967)	55-item checklist of children's behavior
Eyberg Child Behavior Inventory (ECBI)	Eyberg & Ross (1978); Robinson, Eyberg, & Ross (1980)	36-item measure of common child behavior problems. Yields two scores: Intensity and Problem
Conners Parent Rating Scale (CPRS)	Goyette, Conners, & Ulrich (1978)	48-item measure that discriminates between normal and hyperactive children
Abbreviated Conners Parent–Teacher Rating Scale	Conners (1973)	10-item version of the CPRS/Conners Teacher Rating Scale (CTRS)
Home Situations Questionnaire	Barkley (1981); Barkley & Edelbrock (1987)	Measure of specific situations in which behavior problems occur
Werry-Weiss-Peters Activity Rating Scale	Werry & Sprague (1968)	22-item measure of children's hyperactive behavior
SNAP	Pelham, Atkins, Murphy, & White (1981)	23-item checklist criteria for attention deficit disorder (ADD) of the *Diagnostic and Statistical Manual of Mental Disorders;* third edition (DSM-III)
Homework Problem Checklist	Anesko & O'Leary (1983); Shoiock (1978)	20-item measure of the frequency of homework problems during a 2-week period
Conflict Behavior Questionnaire	Prinz et al. (1979)	20-item forced-choice measure of parent-adolescent communication and conflict behavior
Issues Checklist	Prinz et al. (1979)	44-item measure of the frequency and anger intensity of specific parent–adolescent conflict areas
CDI, Parent's Version	Kovacs (1983); Kovacs & Beck (1977)	27-item measure of children's depression
Social Skills Rating System	Gresham & Elliott (in press)	Measure of social skills for children and adolescents aged 3–16. Includes the following factors: Cooperation, Assertion, Responsibility, and Self-Control

TABLE 3.5. *(continued)*

Inventory	References	Content
Teacher report		
CBCL Teacher Report	Achenbach & Edelbrock (1983, 1986)	120-item checklist of a wide variety of behavior problems for children and adolescents aged 6–16
CTRS	Goyette et al. (1978)	28-item measure of hyperactive behaviors
Abbreviated Conners Parent-Teacher Rating Scale	Conners (1973)	10-item version of the CPRS/CTRS
SNAP	Pelham et al. (1981)	23-item checklist of the DSM-II criteria for ADD
Sutter-Eyberg Behavior Inventory	Funderburk & Eyberg (1989)	36-item checklist of common school behavior problems
Social Skills Rating System	Gresham & Elliott (in press)	Measure of social skills for children and adolescents aged 3–16. Includes the following factors: Cooperation, Assertion, and Self-Control
Parent self-report		
Dyadic Adjustment Scale	Spanier (1976)	32-item measure of marital adjustment. Includes four subscales: Dyadic Satisfaction, Dyadic Cohesion, Dyadic Adjustment, and Affectional Expression
Mothers' Activity Checklist	Kelley & Carper (1988)	100-item measure of mothers' pleasant and unpleasant setting events
BDI	Beck et al. (1961)	21-item measure of depression for adolescents and adults (aged 12 and above)
Family Environment Scale	Moos & Moos (1976, 1983)	90-item forced-choice measure of family relationships

In instances where the child's behavior problems include inattentiveness and disruptiveness, I also suggest that parents and teachers complete one or two measures of ADHD, such as the abbreviated or long version of the Conners Parent or Teacher Rating Scale (Conners, 1973; Goyette, Conners, & Ulrich, 1978). However, scores must be interpreted cautiously, as numerous sources of norms and versions of the measures exist (Edelbrock, 1988).

A variety of other paper-and-pencil measures may be appropriate, depending on the situation. Particularly in cases where a parent as opposed to a teacher has initiated contact with the consultant, additional measures of marital adjustment, maternal depression, and family functioning are useful screening tools. In situations where the teacher or school has requested the consultant's assistance, parents often resist completing questionnaires that focus on the family. In such instances, screening for family problems usually is best accomplished in a private interview with the parents. Several measures tapping family or parent dysfunction are described in Table 3.5.

Requiring older children and adolescents to complete measures assessing internalizing disorders can be a helpful adjunct to the interview. When relevant, I assess for depression, negative self-evaluation, and anxiety problems through the use of short questionnaires and the CBCL Youth Self-Report (Achenbach & Edelbrock, 1987). As depression is a relatively common contributor to poor academic performance, I often include a measure of depression as a standard part of the assessment of an adolescent or a child who is at risk for the problem because of recent negative life changes.

In addition to the measures briefly described in Table 3.5, numerous other measures exist that may be of use to the practitioner. For a detailed discussion on the use of questionnaires in the assessment of children, the reader is referred to Edelbrock (1988); Mash and Terdal (1988); and Witt, Cavell, Heffer, Carey, and Martens (1988).

Direct Observation*

Direct observation of a child's behavior is often necessary to conduct a complete behavioral assessment. Many sources have recommended direct observation as a measure of both academic skills and classroom behavior (Alessi, 1988; Shapiro & Lentz, 1986). Because teacher and parent reports may vary, and because such reports may not always be accurate, it is important to obtain a direct, objective sample of the student's behavior.

Direct classroom observation serves several useful functions. The data generated may be used as an important assessment tool; they may also provide a baseline level of performance from which to measure treatment change. For example, if Mary is performing poorly in math, it is important to identify the specific problem. In order to

*The direct observation, other sources of data, and summary sections were written by Dr. Laura Carper.

develop a functional analysis and treatment program, the consultant must be able to assess whether Mary's difficulty in math is the result of poor work habits (which may consist of off-task behavior and in-attentiveness) or the result of a skills deficit in the subject area. Direct observation of Mary in the classroom can determine whether she is using classwork time effectively and attending to material presented by the teacher.

Several standardized codes are available for use in the classroom (e.g., O'Leary, Romanczyk, Kass, Dietz, & Santogrossi, 1979; Saudargas, 1982). The consultant may wish to use an existing code, or may develop a less formal code that can be adapted to varying settings. In many cases, particularly when one is monitoring the presence or absence of a specific behavior, an interval coding system may prove useful. With this type of system, one monitors specific behavior for short intervals, such as 10 or 15 seconds. The observer simply indicates whether or not the behavior occurred during each interval of time. Because there are a consistent number of observations within a specific time period (e.g., twenty 15-second intervals in a 5-minute period of time), it is possible to compare different observation periods throughout the school day.

Shapiro and Lentz (1986) have suggested that certain types of behavioral data are particularly helpful in formulating the student's problem. For example, an estimate of the on-task behavior of the student should be provided. "On-task" behavior consists of any appropriate goal-directed behavior compatible with completing classwork (such as actively working on an assignment or listening to the teacher's presentation of material). "Off-task" behavior therefore consists of behaviors that may compete with or be incompatible with on-task behavior (such as talking to other students or being out of seat). Direct measures of on-task behavior can also be used in conjunction with work samples. For example, in addition to examining Mary's attentiveness, the consultant can also monitor the number of math problems she completes correctly within the class period. This information will be particularly useful in developing a functional analysis; for example, the consultant may find that during class periods in which Mary exhibits a higher percentage of on-task behavior, she also completes a greater number of problems correctly. If the consultant were to monitor work completion or accuracy alone, this relationship might not be evident. Disruptive behavior in the classroom may be monitored with a coding system identical to the one used for on-task behavior. Generally speaking, however, it is best to monitor and target positive child behaviors.

Another student behavior that may prove to be important in developing a treatment program is compliance with the teacher's instructions. This behavior may be computed on a percentage basis, whereby the number of instructions obeyed is divided by the total number of instructions. Compliance may be assessed in a variety of settings, such as the classroom, cafeteria, and playground. In this way, the consultant may determine whether noncompliance (if it exists) is a general problem, or one that pertains specifically to the classroom setting. Finally, teacher behaviors directed toward the student (such as praising or reprimanding) should be monitored as well. The specific behaviors to be monitored in each student's case should be dictated by the information obtained in the teacher interview.

In addition to obtaining observational data on a student's classroom behavior, the assessment process may involve a comparison of the target student with other students in the classroom. This may be achieved by comparing, for example, the target student's on-task time with the on-task time of a randomly selected peer. This information may be useful in distinguishing students who are capable of performing the work but are simply engaged in other behaviors from students who are putting forth a valiant effort but are not able to master the material. For example, if the consultant finds that both Joe and Frank are engaged in on-task behavior approximately 80% of the time, but Joe's work completion and accuracy rates in language are much higher than Frank's, this may suggest that Frank has a specific language skills deficit that may require remediation.

Direct observation may also be helpful in assessing the home environment. This may be desirable when target behaviors involve the completion of homework, for example. Again, the simple on-task versus off-task designation may be informative, as well as a rate of compliance with parental instruction. These behaviors may be monitored using the same type of coding systems described for classroom behavior. Several standardized home observation codes are available if more complex information is sought (e.g., Forehand & McMahon, 1981; Wahler, House, & Stambaugh, 1976). Other types of information that may prove valuable, particularly in monitoring homework progress, include rates of work completion and accuracy.

Generally, direct observation is best utilized when the student is of elementary school age. Older children may react more negatively to the presence of the observer. In addition, older children are more likely to be exhibiting behaviors that are not necessary or possible to observe (truancy, tardiness). It is always best to consider the specific problems identified by the teachers and parents in deciding whether direct observation is warranted.

Other Sources of Data

In addition to direct observation, a variety of other sources of data may prove to be helpful in the assessment process. School records, for example, contain a wealth of information about a student's past performance that may aid in the assessment process. Some of this information may include results of standardized testing, achievement scores, past grades, absences or truancy, rule violations, suspensions, detentions, and teacher evaluations. For example, this information may be helpful in determining whether the current problem has been progressing for some time or is a recent development. The pattern of deterioration is important, since a sudden decrease in achievement or increase in problem behavior may signal that the student is experiencing some type of emotional or physical distress. Achievement test data may prove very useful as well; these scores indicate whether the student is functioning at a level commensurate with his or her age and grade. So, for instance, if a student's achievement scores are on grade level or above, and his or her grades are poor, the problem is probably a performance deficit rather than a skills deficit. The type of information contained in the school record serves as a type of academic history of the student. For this reason, reviewing it should be a routine part of the assessment process.

The student himself or herself also may be called upon to provide additional assessment data. Self-monitoring of class attendance, on-task behavior, homework completion, or the like may provide the consultant with supplementary data about the student's behavior. For example, the daily report card itself may be used as a source of self-monitored data. An older student in particular may be allowed to complete the card with respect to such behavior as attendance or work completion. The teacher can then check the card for accuracy. In this way, the student provides information about himself or herself to both the parents and teacher.

Self-monitoring gives students immediate feedback about their behavior, and may also provide the consultant with the students' view or evaluation of their own behavior. The procedure may be used to increase self-awareness (Shapiro, 1988). For example, the consultant may want to include a place on the report card for students to evaluate themselves, using a question such as "Did you try your best today?" or "How was your motivation today?" This type of self-feedback may serve to help the students remember that they are in control of their own behavior.

SUMMARY

Behavioral assessment is a practical, empirically based approach to assessing school and home functioning. Particularly valuable characteristics of behavioral assessment include its emphasis on specifying behavior excesses and deficits, the molecular level of the assessment, and the relatively low level of inference compared to traditional assessment. A primary feature of behavioral assessment is that it is a hypothesis-testing process that leads directly to problem solving. This establishes a link between the assessment and treatment processes. The major theoretical basis of behavioral methods of assessment is found in behavior analysis. Behavior analysis is concerned with identifying the many possible antecedents and consequences of a given behavior, and the effects that these antecedents and consequences may have on that behavior. I consider the functional analysis of behavior to be an essential tool in effective clinical practice.

Other assessment considerations include direct assessment of academic skills using criterion-referenced assessment, focusing on both the child's current skill level and the environmental variables associated with academic performance. A myriad of student, teacher, and family variables may also affect children's school performance. Being sensitive to these variables is an important part of the assessment (and treatment) process as well.

Among the most important assessment procedures in developing a functional analysis are behavioral consultation interviews. These interviews focus on problem identification, problem analysis, and problem evaluation. Additional assessment procedures that may provide valuable information include paper-and-pencil instruments, direct observation of classroom behavior, and other sources of academic data such as school records. Behavior analysis involves the combination of all types of information about the child, his or her family, and the classroom setting that contribute to the maintenance of the problem behavior. If this analysis is done properly, the development of the treatment program should be a logical extension of the assessment process.

APPENDIX 3.1
Child Intake Form for Use in a Parent Interview

CHILD INTAKE

Name _____   Date _____

School _____   Teacher/Grade _____

DEVELOPMENTAL HISTORY:

Cognitive Milestones Reached:	On time	Early	Delayed
Motor Milestones Reached:	On time	Early	Delayed

Describe any problems _____

_____

Medical history:

Ear/Respiratory Infections   Hospitalizations   Operations
Medications   High Fevers   Hearing/Visual Impairments   Other

Elaborate if circled _____

_____

Traumatic life events:

Parent's Divorce/Remarriage   Death of Family Member   New School
Sexual/Physical Abuse   Legal Problems   Other

Elaborate if circled _____

Early childhood history:

Noncompliant   Aggressive   Fearful   Impulsive   Poor Social Skills
Excessively Active   Socially Isolated   Other

Elaborate if circled _____

_____

CURRENT FAMILY FUNCTIONING:

Noncompliance:	Chores Routines (morning/bedtime) Other
Delinquent Behaviors:	Fighting Stealing Lying Arguing Drug Use
Social Difficulties:	Few Friends Poor Social Skills Aggressive

From *School–Home Notes: Promoting Children's Classroom Success* by Mary Lou Kelley. © 1990 The Guilford Press.

Homework Completion: Stalls   Sloppy   Argumentative
Disorganized   Fails to bring assign-
ments home/back to school

Hyperactive Behaviors: Excessively active   Impulsive
Inattentive

Toileting problems: Enuresis   Encopresis

Other: _____

Elaborate if circled _____

Parent and family history:

Marital Distress   Legal Problems   Alcohol/Drug Abuse   Depression
Psychiatric Problems   Job-Related Difficulties   Financial Difficulties
Poor Social Support/Insularity   Other

Elaborate if Circled _____

_____

Child's relationship with:

Mother:	Excellent	Good	Fair	Poor
Father:	Excellent	Good	Fair	Poor
Siblings:	Excellent	Good	Fair	Poor

Parenting discipline methods:

Spanking   Time Out   Praise/Rewards   Response Cost
Clear Instructions   Discussion   Other

Describe _____

_____

Spouse Consistency in Disciplining: Excellent   Good   Fair   Poor
Spouse Support in Disciplining and
Caretaking: Excellent   Good   Fair   Poor
Support from Other Household
Members: Excellent   Good   Fair   Poor

Elaborate _____

_____

Types of rewards available at home:

TV   VCR Movie   Activity with Friend   Activity with Parent
Stickers   Special Food Item   Money   Other

Elaborate _____

_____

Other Pertinent Child or Family History or Current Functioning:_____

_____

_____

_____

ACADEMIC HISTORY AND CURRENT FUNCTIONING

Schools Attended: _____

_____

_____

Special Conditions:

    Failed Grades   Special Placement   Suspensions   Other

Elaborate if circled _____

_____

_____

CURRENT ACADEMIC AND CLASSROOM FUNCTIONING:

Current Achievement Scores:

Math:	Below Average	Average	Above Average
Reading:	Below Average	Average	Above Average

Current Grades:

Math	_____	Science	_____
Reading	_____	Soc Studies	_____
English	_____	Other	_____

School Problems:

    Academic Skills: Poor Work Completion   Daydreams/Inattentive
                      Fails to Bring Homework   Careless

                      Other _____

    Behavior in Class: Aggressiveness   Talking   Out of seat
                      Doesn't Follow rules   Withdrawn

                      Other _____

Elaborate if circled _____

_____

Discipline Used at School:

    Point System   Reprimands   Time Out   Removal of privileges
    Punishment Work   Daily Note   Other

Elaborate if circled _____

_____

Relationship with Teacher:

    Teacher–Child Relationship: Excellent   Good   Fair   Poor
    Teacher–Parent Relationship: Excellent   Good   Fair   Poor

Elaborate if needed _____

_____

ACCEPTABILITY OF SCHOOL-HOME NOTE SYSTEM:

    Teacher: Good   Fair   Poor   Parent: Good   Fair   Poor

If poor, describe _____

_____

_____

_____

_____

OTHER INFORMATION ABOUT ACADEMIC HISTORY OR CURRENT BEHAVIOR

_____

_____

_____

_____

_____

TREATMENT GOALS FOR HOME/SCHOOL

_____

_____

_____

4

Developing and Using School–Home Notes

The literature review presented in Chapter 2 attests to the effectiveness of school–home notes. The procedure has been shown to improve a variety of behavior problems exhibited by children ranging from preschoolers to high school students. Daily report cards have been used to reduce inappropriate classroom behavior, to improve academic skill acquisition, and to increase work completion. The procedure has worked to improve children's behavior even in the most lax of treatment conditions: School–home notes have been effective when target behaviors, treatment goals, and contingencies of reinforcement were vaguely specified and when parents and teachers received very little training in administering the procedure. Given the apparent robustness and versatility of school–home notes, does it matter how they are designed, implemented, and evaluated? Are there circumstances in which daily report cards are more likely to be effective than in others?

I believe that the answer is yes. True, the literature does not strongly support the superiority of a single treatment package; daily report cards apparently often work in vaguely defined circumstances. However, many of the studies reviewed employed the procedure with nonclinical samples. In contrast, the realities of clinical practice and treatment of over 80 children suggest that some school–home note programs are more likely to produce significant, socially valid changes in behavior than are many alternative interventions.

The vast majority of *clinical* uses of school–home notes are directed toward modifying the behavior of a single child, rather than that of entire classrooms of students. To warrant referral to a consultant, the child probably exhibits behavior problems throughout the school day rather than during a single class period. The child may not be completing classwork or may be behaving disruptively. The referred child probably exhibits both academic and conduct problems, as in the case of Timothy presented in Chapter 1.

Assuming that this typical child could potentially benefit from a school–home note program (as indicated by the consultant's functional analysis), my colleagues and I recommend incorporating a number of features into the procedure. For example, unlike the subjects in the daily report card programs described in the literature, most clinical cases exhibit behavior that requires monitoring and treatment throughout the school day rather than during a single period. If this is to be accomplished, the recording procedure must be easy for teachers to use and for parents to comprehend. Target responses should be clearly specified, so that parents, teachers, and children are aware of the criteria for satisfactory performance. The consequences for appropriate behavior must be sufficiently potent to compete with the powerful influence of peer attention for inappropriate behavior. Finally, parents and teachers must be trained adequately in contingency management techniques to employ the procedure in a positive, consistent manner. When these features are missing, it is likely that the school–home note program will not be implemented with integrity and/or will not be effective.

This chapter focuses on the mechanics of setting up an effective school–home program. The chapter is broken down into four major sections: setting the stage for effective parent–teacher communication; designing the school–home note program; establishing contingencies for satisfactory performance; and implementing treatment. The suggestions presented in this chapter and Chapter 5 are based on the critique of the literature presented in Chapter 2, on clinical experience, and on a strong belief in the application of behavioral principles to understanding and changing children's behavior. Summaries and examples of recommended practices are provided in the appendices at the end of this chapter in the form of parent/teacher handouts and sample school–home notes.

SETTING THE STAGE

In this section, the ways of laying the foundation for successful use of a school–home note program are described. Specifically, the consultant should address four issues prior to using the procedure: (1) determine whether a child is an appropriate candidate for the procedure; (2) promote parent and teacher cooperation with the procedure; (3) introduce the school-home note concept; and (4) select members of the school-home team.

Selecting Appropriate Clients

As indicated in Chapter 3, school–home notes are not appropriate for all children. Children who have very severe behavior problems or academic deficits, or who come from highly dysfunctional families, may not be helped by the program. Use of school–home notes in these circumstances may only accentuate the need for alternative placement or more comprehensive treatment. The school–home note treatment could cause further deterioration in parent–teacher communication or increase punitive parental behavior toward the child.

The program may also be ineffective when a child needs more frequent and immediate consequences than are normally included in a school–home note program. The amelioration of a child's behavior problems may require the use of in-class contingency management procedures, such as those used in a token economy. Some children may require immediate removal from the situation where they have behaved inappropriately.

For obvious reasons, school–home notes should not be considered when teachers or parents balk at participating in the program. My colleagues and I have encountered cases in which consultees resisted using the procedure in spite of its apparent appropriateness and the presentation of normally persuasive rationales. In these instances, we suggest that alternative solutions be generated, regardless of how well a daily reporting system *might* work. The intervention will not be used with integrity if the potential treatment consumers view it as unacceptable.

Although school–home notes are not appropriate in all situations and are not well received by all parents and teachers, we have found the treatment to be a useful adjunctive intervention in most circumstances. In situations where motivation affects performance and/or children can benefit from increased parental involvement in the learning process, use of daily report cards normally produces many positive consequences. For example, the notes often result in more positive interactions among parents, teachers, and the child; improved classroom behavior; and diminished parent and teacher frustration with the child and his or her behavior.

School–home notes also can be helpful in informing parents about a child's progress in alternative therapies. For example, if the child is participating in a special reading program, school–home notes can be used to inform parents about the child's reading productivity and skill acquisition. Thus, daily report cards are useful whenever feedback to parents and increased parental involvement in the educational process may serve to promote children's social and academic development.

With regard to using school–home notes with children of various ages, my colleagues and I have effectively used the procedure with children as young as 3 and as old as 16. The consultant should be sensitive to young children's language and cognitive abilities, as well as to their responsivity to delayed reinforcement. With young children, we often use a school–home note system along with in-class contingency management procedures. For example, a note used with a young preschooler for decreasing aggressive, noncompliant behavior during preschool is shown in Figure 4.1. The note is simple and the evaluation criteria are depicted by happy, neutral, and sad faces rather than by words. The procedure, which coupled home and

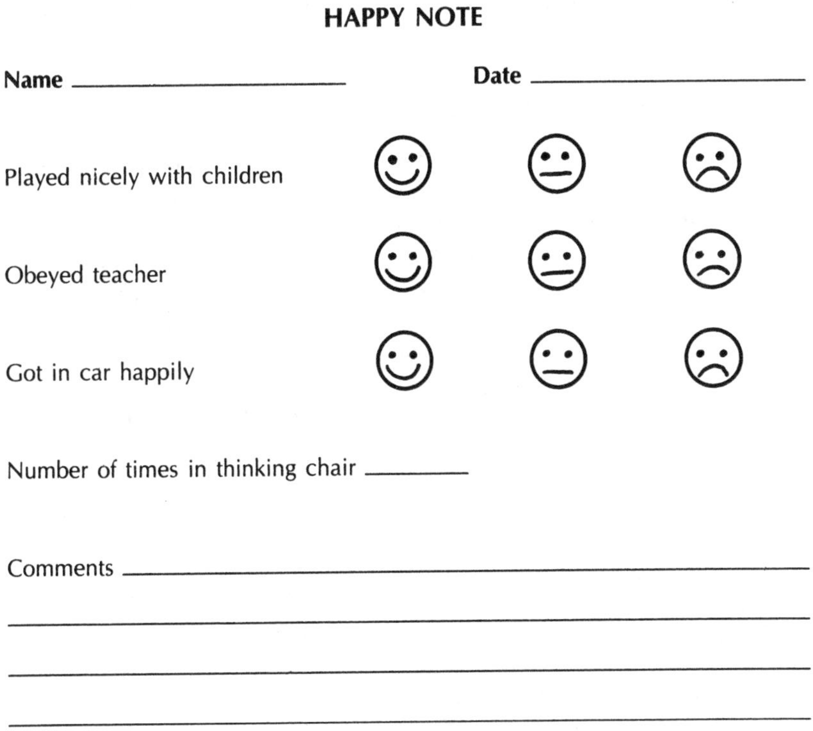

HAPPY NOTE

Name ____________________ **Date** ____________________

Played nicely with children

Obeyed teacher

Got in car happily

Number of times in thinking chair ________

Comments ____

FIGURE 4.1. School–home note used with an aggressive, oppositional preschooler.

school contingency management procedures, was effective in increasing the child's appropriate behavior. The school program consisted of time out for inappropriate behavior and praise for appropriate behavior. Importantly, these procedures alone were ineffective prior to beginning the school–home program.

If parents have control over potent reinforcers, school–home notes can be as effective with adolescents as with younger children. However, given the possibility of peer ridicule, the procedure with adolescents should be used judiciously and with respect for the teenagers' feelings. Some adolescents greatly resist the idea of using a school–home note system, because they view the procedure as childish or dislike the idea of increased parental involvement in their school life. Many times, however, teenagers view the procedure as a welcome change to constant nagging from parents about schoolwork. Thus, the consultant should not assume that an adolescent will resist the treatment just because it is more often used with younger children. (Methods of increasing adolescents' cooperation with a school–home note system, including modifications in the standard format, are discussed later in this book.)

Promoting Parent and Teacher Cooperation

Perhaps the greatest contribution the consultant can make to promoting parent and teacher cooperation is to assume the role of neutral mediator and child advocate. Usually the consultant is contacted by *either* the parent or the teacher and presented with a description of the child's behavior problems. Rather than simply aligning ourselves with that person, however, my colleagues and I involve both teachers and parents early in the assessment process and attempt to take a neutral position. For example, we often see families who initiate assistance because of their concern over their children's unsatisfactory academic progress. Although parents sometimes express dissatisfaction with a teacher's approach to problem solving, we usually maintain a neutral stance and encourage parents to adapt a more positive approach. We describe the benefits of a team approach to problem solving and suggest that the teacher be given ample opportunity to participate in assessment and treatment. Then, with the parents' permission, the teacher is contacted and asked to participate in the assessment.

It often is best to interview parents and teachers separately at least once during the assessment. We use this opportunity to obtain a history and gather information pertinent to the functional analysis. Private interviews give parents and teachers an opportunity to freely discuss problems they have encountered with each other and to reveal information about the child or family that they would otherwise withhold. For example, a parent may discuss his or her belief that the teacher only wants the child in another class or on medication and probably will be unwilling to work to solve the problem. The teacher may provide information about the parents' lack of consistent follow-through with previous programs, or may discuss issues of family dysfunction revealed to her by the child.

To be an effective mediator, the consultant should assure parents and teachers that all information provided will be kept confidential and will be used only for the purposes of planning treatment. Of course, the consultant must adhere to the legal mandates of P.L. 94-142 and other laws regarding the treatment of minors. Generally, rules involving children promote parental involvement in the assessment and treatment process. We suggest going beyond the legal requirements to more active encouragement of team participation early in the assessment process.

Introducing the School–Home Note Concept

The sessions conducted individually with parents and teachers are useful for establishing rapport and showing support. The individual sessions also can be used to introduce school–home notes as a possible treatment method. When discussing school–home notes for the first time, the consultant should present a clear rationale and explanation of the procedure. Such a presentation should include (1) a brief description of the procedure and the roles of the school–home note team members (parents, teacher, child, and consultant); (2) the benefits of a team approach to problem solving including enhanced parent–teacher communication; and (3) the advantages of home-based as opposed to school-based reinforcement procedures. These advantages must be tailored to the particular situation, but may include the greater availability of rewards in the home and the minimal time required of the teacher to administer the program.

It is also recommended that the topic of school–home notes be introduced within an empathetic context. For example, the consultant could introduce the concept of a school–home note to a teacher by saying something like the following:

> "Mrs. Smith, it seems that to some extent Timothy's problems are due to his not trying to do his best. At times he appears to put forth little effort to complete his work or behave appropriately. He seems to be a more difficult child to manage than most of your other students. I see that the

procedures which normally work have not been very effective for you; his disruptive behavior is difficult to manage in a classroom setting. You really are going to need some help dealing with him.

"One procedure that I have used in the past, which may improve Timothy's behavior without taking up an undue amount of your time, is a school–home note system. The procedure involves a teacher's evaluating a child's behavior daily. The child's parents are responsible for rewarding the child for good behavior and using the feedback to teach the child how to behave appropriately. My role would be to assist in problem solving and facilitate communication.

"Many teachers with whom we have worked have found the program to be minimally time-consuming and very helpful. We often find that the procedure helps build positive communication between parents and teachers. In Timothy's case, the program might be particularly helpful in letting the parents know about the school day and all the things you do to help Timothy improve his behavior. They probably will feel that they are participating more fully in Timothy's education, and this should help them feel less frustrated.

"I realize there are a lot of specifics to work out. I will need to know exactly which aspects of Timothy's behavior you consider most problematic. I also realize that we would need to design a school–home note system that could be easily incorporated into your routine. Assuming that this could be done, how do you feel in general about using school–home notes with Timothy?"

In this example, the consultant empathizes with the difficulty of the teacher's job and avoids being critical of the teacher or Timothy's parents. As recommended by Bergan (1977), the consultant also summarizes the problems of concern and avoids discussing the etiology of the unacceptable behavior. The possible use of a school–home note system is brought up directly, although the consultant emphasizes the teacher's important role in determining whether the procedure is appropriate and encourages her involvement in designing Timothy's program.

After introducing the idea to teachers and parents, the consultant should provide them with some examples of notes that have been used in the past with other children. Assuming that the adults agree to consider using the procedure, the consultant should provide them with the handout shown in Appendix 4.1; ask them to read over the material; and schedule a team conference. The handout is intended for both parents and teachers and describes the activities involved in designing and using the school–home note procedure. For the reader's convenience, the handout is briefly summarized in Table 4.1.

TABLE 4.1. Version of "Home-Based Rewards for Classroom Behavior: Use of School–Home Notes" (See Appendix 4.1)

Steps in Designing and Using a School-Home Note Program

1. *Conduct a parent–teacher conference.*

   At this meeting teachers, parents, and other relevant individuals should discuss what they consider to be acceptable and desirable behavior and what behaviors the child displays that are problematic. Both teachers and parents should avoid blaming and should try to make their discussion as pleasant as possible.

2. *Define target behaviors.*

   Using the information discussed, the team members should define specific, observable target behaviors. They should emphasize behaviors that are worded positively, occur frequently, and are directly relevant to academic performance.

3. *Set small, clearly defined goals.*

   Children's performance should be evaluated at frequent intervals throughout the day. In this way, small changes in behavior can be detected and rewarded. When requiring improved performance, team members should set small goals that are clearly within the child's ability to achieve. Parents, teachers, and students should be well aware of the criteria for goal achievement.

4. *Design the school–home note.*

   Each note should have a place for the child's name, the date, each teacher's signature, and comments.

5. *Establish responsibilities.*

   Before starting the school–home note program, the teachers, parents, and child should meet to establish each person's responsibilities. It should be a teacher's responsibility to provide the child with a completed note each day. The parents are responsible for rewarding desirable behaviors.

6. *Determine rewards.*

   With the help of the child, the team should decide on a set of daily and weekly rewards that are provided for satisfactory performance.

7. *Explain the note.*

   In a positive manner, the team should tell the child that the program is intended to help him or her do better in school and improve his or her relationship with teachers and parents.

8. *Collect baseline data.*

   The teachers should complete the note for about a week without providing rewards for improved classwork or behavior. Baseline data provide information for setting up specific target behaviors and determining small, fair goals for earning rewards. During baseline, parents can reward the child for simply bringing the completed note home.

TABLE 4.1. *(continued)*

9. *Provide feedback.*

   School–home notes work best when teachers and parents provide frequent verbal feedback and praise. Teachers should notice and praise appropriate behavior frequently throughout the day. Parents should review the daily note and comment on the child's performance.

10. *Provide promised consequences.*

   It is very important to follow through with promised consequences each time the child brings home a school–home note that meets the daily goal for a reward.

11. *Fade the note when behavior improves.*

   As behavior improves, the school–home note system should be faded out. A good way to do this is to shift to longer evaluation intervals. For example, a child can be evaluated two times a day rather than six. Later, notes can be faded to use on a weekly basis.

As shown in Table 4.1, the steps to setting up an effective school–home note system begin with arranging a parent–teacher conference and conclude with fading out the procedure as behavior improves. The handout delineates the responsibilities of program participants and encourages the use of positive communication behavior focusing on problem solving. When parents and teachers are provided with the handout prior to the conference, they can familiarize themselves with the program and develop a better understanding of their role in the treatment process. In addition, parents and teachers are able to make a more informed decision about whether they view a daily report card system as an appropriate and potentially effective intervention.

Selecting the Team Members

The school–home note team should include all adults who will be involved in administering the intervention or who may contribute to its success by supporting program participants. Of course, parents and teachers are essential members of the school–home note team, and it is always important to actively involve both in the assessment and treatment process. However, other school officials or family members may be helpful to include in the school–home note conference. The consultant, in collaboration with the parent and teacher, should carefully consider who should be involved in the program for it to be effective. For example, it may be that the child does the majority of his or her homework after school with a babysitter while the mother is at work. If so, the babysitter should attend the conferences, or at least should be considered an important member of the school–home note team and given the opportunity to provide input into the program.

Various school personnel should be considered as potential members of the school–home note team. Their inclusion depends on the organization of the school and the specific child. When children have several teachers, as is the case with most junior high or high school students, guidance counselors can greatly facilitate communication among teachers. A good guidance counselor can be very helpful in monitoring the program and dealing with routine questions from teachers. In fact, with proper training, many guidance counselors can set up and monitor school–home note programs. For example, my colleagues and I worked with an interested and skilled junior high school counselor who, after participating on two school–home note teams, began to use the procedure routinely with unmotivated students. She competently enlisted parent and teacher cooperation and effectively administered the program. With many children, she used the school–home note shown (in an abbreviated form) in Figure 4.2. The note in Figure 4.2 was completed by several of Richard's teachers and his parents. (Other daily notes are provided in Appendix 4.2.)

Other school personnel may be appropriate to include on a school–home note team; if they are not included, the consultant may at least wish to inform them about his or her work with the child and to enlist their support. Depending on the organization of the school and the behavior problems exhibited by the child, these school employees might include the school principal or vice-principal; a teacher's aide; the child's bus driver; and support/special education personnel, such as the child's speech or physical therapist.

With regard to the home environment, it may be helpful to include any number of different family members or child caretakers on the school–home note team. It is strongly recommended that both parents attend the school–home note conference in order to promote spouse consistency. Even in situations where the parents are divorced, we encourage some level of involvement in the program by the noncustodial parent whenever appropriate. For example, we sometimes suggest that the custodial parent provide the ex-spouse with the handout and a copy of the child's school–home note, as well as encourage some level of participation. The noncustodial parent may be responsible for providing daily or weekly rewards when these are earned by the child on his or her visitation days. Other individuals who may be valuable team members include afternoon babysitters (as noted above) or relatives with whom the child frequently visits.

It is not necessary for every team member to attend school–home

SCHOOL–HOME NOTE

Name ___Richard___   **Date** ___10/20___

SUBJECT___Math___

Was prepared for class	(Yes) No NA	Homework assignment:
Used class time well	(Yes) No NA	Test Friday on
Handed in homework	(Yes) No NA	Chapter 3

Homework/(Test)Grade   F D (C) B A NA   Teacher's Initials _WJ_

Comments: Seems to be paying attention better and using his time well.

___

SUBJECT___Social Studies___

Was prepared for class	Yes (No) NA	Homework assignment:
Used class time well	(Yes) No NA	Answer questions
Handed in homework	Yes (No) NA	1–10, page 113

(Homework)Test Grade   F (D) C B A NA   Teacher's Initials _MS_

Comments: Did not bring notebook; he talked a good bit during class.

___

SUBJECT___English___

Was prepared for class	(Yes) No NA	Homework assignment:
Used class time well	(Yes) No NA	None
Handed in homework	Yes No (NA)	

Homework(Test)Grade   F D (C) B A NA   Teacher's Initials _TL_

Comments: Participated nicely in class.

___

Parent Comments: ___Ms. Sessions, Richard says he handed in his___

___homework. Would you mind checking with him?___

FIGURE 4.2. Abbreviated school–home note used with middle and high school students. (This note was completed by Richard, his teachers, and his parents.)

note conferences. Involving a large number of individuals in designing the school–home note would be unwieldy. However, all relevant parties should be encouraged to provide input and should be given the understanding that they are an important part of the school–home note team. Attendance at the conference should be based on the expected level of involvement of each team member in the program.

DESIGNING THE SCHOOL–HOME NOTE PROGRAM

This section describes the specific tasks involved in designing a school–home note program. The activities are presented in sufficient detail to allow the consultant who is unfamiliar with them to design an effective program. The consultant may find that certain procedures can be abbreviated as he or she becomes accustomed to developing and administering the treatment. For example, a consultant may be able to define target behaviors and construct the note primarily through consulting by telephone with the teacher and providing him or her with handouts. We strongly recommend, however, that the suggestions provided below be followed and not circumvented for the sake of time efficiency by consultants inexperienced in using the school–home note program.

The following activities usually take place across at least two different sessions that are attended by selected members of the school–home note team. The sessions are generally attended by both a parent and the teacher. The goals of the first team conference usually parallel those of the problem analysis interview described in Chapter 3; the session emphasizes identifying and operationalizing specific problem behaviors, as well as designing and beginning treatment. The second conference generally focuses on evaluating treatment outcome and refining the intervention. This conference basically accomplishes the goals of the problem evaluation interview discussed in Chapter 3.

Providing an Overview

At the beginning of the school–home note conference, the consultant should review the content of previous discussions with team members, including rationales for using a school–home note system and should specify the tasks to be accomplished during the conference. The consultant's introductory remarks set the stage for positive, cooperative interactions among team members, and should be carefully and sensitively worded. It often is best to assume that both parents and teachers are going to be at least a little defensive about their prior attempts at problem solving. Thus, the consultant should avoid comments that may accentuate this defensiveness and should use facilitative, complimentary statements. For example, the consultant should avoid referring to past errors in judgment and instead should emphasize instances where each party has put forth effort toward remediating the child's problem behavior.

In summarizing past discussions, the consultant should attempt to guide the conversation in ways that promote productive problem solving. In particular, discussions about the child's problem behavior should be couched in objective, specific terms and descriptions. For example, the consultant may say, "All of us are concerned that Jenny is not completing her classwork on a consistent basis in the time allotted," as opposed to "Jenny's biggest problem seems to be that we just cannot get her to pay attention to what is going on in the classroom. She just seems to get lost in her thoughts." As shown in this example, value-laden statements that presumably describe inherent qualities of the child should be avoided; they are distracting and unlikely to foster problem solving.

Defining and providing a rationale for adopting a school–home note program should consist of a brief and general presentation. The consultant should distribute copies of the handouts to team members and succinctly describe the format of the procedure. He or she should remind the participants of the general activities involved in setting up a school–home note system, and should review the rationales for using the procedure with the specific child. This presentation helps to insure that team members are equally familiar with the program and hold similar expectations of one another.

It is important that team members be encouraged to ask questions and voice concerns about the school–home note program. As participants express their opinions, other treatment alternatives may surface, or a team member may develop misgivings about the school–home procedure. The consultant should attempt to address these concerns thoroughly and to remain open-minded about treatment. If the procedure is judged to be unacceptable by a team member, then it is unlikely to be used with integrity or used at all (Witt, Elliott, Gresham, & Kramer, 1988). After addressing the concerns, however, the consultant should continue with the next step toward problem solving—defining target behaviors—prior to dismissing school–home notes as an appropriate treatment. Sometimes the precise nature of the problem is not fully appreciated by team members until the child's behavior excesses and deficits are delineated.

At various points in the assessment and treatment process, parents and teachers may express concern that a school–home note system will not address the child's *real* problems. They may insist, for example, that the child is hyperactive or has a personality problem. These issues often come up during individual discussions with the teacher and parent, or during the consultant's overview of school–home notes. Again, these concerns should be addressed. One approach is to agree that many other things may be going on that contribute to the child's problem, but that a school–home note program may represent a first step toward problem solving. The treatment is easy to implement, and when administered appropriately, often produces changes in behavior relatively quickly. Thus, the "cost" of giving the intervention a good try is small. Alternative interventions, such as medication, placement, or more extensive family or child therapy, generally are more intrusive, restrictive, expensive, and/or permanent.

The following narrative provides an abbreviated example of a consultant's introductory remarks made during a school–home note conference.

"I have talked with most of you about Timothy's problems in school. All of you agree that he is a bright, likeable child who is able to do the work. I have enjoyed my interactions with Timothy and believe he sincerely would like his situation to be more positive.

"Before we get too far into this meeting, I would like to generally review some of the behaviors we would like to see Timothy exhibit, the steps in using a school–home note system, and the reasons why the intervention may be appropriate for Timothy. Please feel free to ask questions and make comments. There are many areas where we will need everyone's ideas to solve the problem most effectively.

"Based on my discussions with each of you, we generally agree that Timothy is quite capable of doing more work but, at this point, refuses to complete his class assignments the majority of the time. This results in Timothy's needing to do a lot of homework, which is a burden on his parents. Timothy clearly needs to work more productively during class time. In addition to classwork, the Warrens would like to improve Timothy's productivity during the homework session. Thus, at both home and school, we would like to see Timothy complete his work with less supervision and in a more appropriate period of time.

"With regard to Timothy's behavior, we would like to work toward helping him behave in a more cooperative, less disruptive manner. We probably will see an improvement in this behavior as he completes more schoolwork. Nonetheless, it is important to get Timothy to raise his hand before talking and to refrain from bothering other children during class time. Part of the problem is that the other children seem to give him a lot of attention when he is disruptive. However, with everyone working together, I hope that we can help Timothy learn to get attention in more appropriate ways.

"I suggest that we consider using a school–home note program to help solve Timothy's problems. The treatment, if we decide to use it, will involve Mrs. Smith's evaluating Timothy's behavior and the Warrens' rewarding Timothy when he behaves satisfactorily. As the handout indicates, we will clearly define the behaviors Timothy should perform more often. Next, we will set performance goals and determine rewards for Timothy to earn when he achieves his goals. We should list privileges that are truly important to Timothy. Should you agree to participate in a school–home note program, everyone will need to be positive with Timothy and work together to help Timothy behave.

"We have discussed a number of reasons for using a school–home note with Timothy. What do each of you think could be gained by using the procedure?. . . Now that we have discussed the positive features of the program, are there any concerns about the program that you have? . . .

"If any concerns arise as we discuss the program or you hit upon any new ideas, please feel free to make comments. Remember, a school–home note has to be something each of you feels good about using, if it is going to work very well. A lot of times, small changes can make a big difference in how easy or how well the procedure works. If you have *any* ideas or concerns, please speak up.

"Before we begin working out the program, let me say that I believe all of you have sincerely tried to help solve Timothy's problems. Helping him behave better has required a great deal of time already. I appreciate your enthusiasm and willingness to try something new after all the work you have already put into helping Timothy. I really believe our efforts will pay off with all of us working together."

Selecting and Defining Target Behaviors

Selecting relevant, socially valid target behaviors is critical to the success of school–home notes. The team members should view the behaviors as important to the child's academic and social success. Unless parents and teachers genuinely value the selected behaviors, they are unlikely to administer the program wholeheartedly.

In general, academic products such as work completion and accuracy should be chosen over "process" behaviors such as remaining on task (Hoge & Andrews, 1987). Parents and teachers usually agree that academic products are important. Behaviors such as rate of work completion can be monitored quickly and objectively by teachers; evaluations of these behaviors can be interpreted easily by parents and children. These qualities will contribute to the continued use of school–home notes by team members.

My colleagues and I recommend that, whenever feasible, target behaviors involving classroom conduct be singled out for treatment only after a period of rewarding academic productivity. The consultant may include social behaviors such as "Did not disturb others during class time" on the school–home note, but should discourage their initial inclusion in the contingency program. Giving priority to academic rather than conduct goals is suggested because children's classroom behavior often improves after rewarding increases in work productivity. Thus, it may prove unnecessary to include classroom conduct goals in the contingency program after obtaining improvements in academic responses.

Although it is generally recommended that the consultant focus on work productivity, there are times when a child's disruptiveness markedly interferes with the classroom routine. In these cases, the teacher may demand or the behavior may require a more direct intervention approach. For example, the teacher may ask to be told how to handle the child's conduct problems, or may request that the child's disruptiveness be included in the treatment. The consultant must be sensitive to the intrusiveness of the child's behavior problems and be responsive to teacher and parent concerns. In situations where intervention efforts are primarily directed toward remediating conduct problems, we suggest that target behaviors relevant to academic productivity should also be included on the school–home note. In this way, the completed note prompts parents and teachers to acknowledge and praise the child for acceptable academic performance.

Before asking team members to provide their own ideas about which behaviors to change, the consultant should discuss the characteristics of a good target behavior and provide examples. This presentation provides consultees with a frame of reference and can expedite the selection of operationally defined target responses. Referring back to the handout (See Appendix 4.1), the consultant should endorse selecting target behaviors that (1) represent academic products rather than process responses; (2) are defined in very specific, observable terms; (3) occur or should occur frequently throughout the school day; (4) can easily be monitored by the teacher; (5) are likely to be sensitive to treatment effects; (6) are judged as important by all team members; and, (7) are worded positively whenever possible. Several examples of target behavior descriptors that do and do not encompass these characteristics are shown in Table 4.2.

The consultant should emphasize the need to define problem behaviors operationally, so that all team members and the child will know when the behavior is to be performed. We have found that this is a particularly difficult task for most consultees. Providing several examples, however, can facilitate their ability to generate concrete definitions of problem behavior and can reduce their use of vague, global problem descriptions. For example, the consultant may say:

> "A good target behavior definition describes the specific observable actions the child must do to perform the behavior. For instance, the target

TABLE 4.2. Examples of Constructive and Less Constructive Target Behavior Descriptors

Recommended	Not Recommended
Percentage of work completed correctly (math, reading, etc.).	Did not complete classwork. Please finish at home.
Used class time well (math, reading, etc.).	Daydreaming.
Talked only with permission.	Disrupted other students.
Prepared for class.	No homework in reading.
Handed in homework (math, reading, etc.).	Earned a happy face today.
Behaved cooperatively before and after class period.	Out of seat, disrupted others.
Obeyed instructions without arguing.	Sassy, disrespectful.
Played nicely with other children.	Fought at recess.
Participated during class.	Did not pay attention during class (math, reading, etc.).

Note. For criteria for defining target behaviors, see text and Appendix 4.1.

behavior definition for 'Prepared for class' might be 'Had two pencils, the appropriate class notebook, and the appropriate book on his desk at the beginning of a class.' "

It is useful to select and define target behaviors that are applicable across an entire school day and whose occurrence can be evaluated at frequent intervals during the day. In this way, the teacher can simply evaluate whether the behavior occurred during a specific time period. For example, using the behavior "Prepared for class," the teacher can evaluate the occurrence of the behavior for each class period. As shown in Table 4.2, other behaviors that are applicable across many situations throughout the school day include "Percentage of classwork completed correctly," "Used class time well," "Participated during class," "Behaved cooperatively before and during class," and "Talked only with permission" for school-age children, and "Obeyed teacher without arguing," "Quiet during nap time," "Followed directions," and "Played nicely without hitting" for preschoolers.

Very often, intervals are distinguished by changes in the child's routine environment (e.g., different class subjects, or the period before vs. the period after lunch). It is frequently the case that a child's behavior is more problematic in some settings than in others. For example, the child may consistently refuse to complete his or her math assignment, but usually participates appropriately in reading group. As behavior may fluctuate across settings, the consultant should attempt to break the day down into naturally occurring time intervals. This allows one to vary performance criteria, depending on baseline performance across situations.

The degree to which children are involved in school–home note conferences should be decided on a case-by-case basis. Usually, the older the child, the more input he or she should have in assisting with the development of their treatment program. The opinions of adolescents should be strongly considered and included in the program. My colleagues and I find that adolescents generally are more cooperative with treatment when they believe their opinions are given proper weight by members of the treatment team. Adolescents often are able to generate ideas about treatment and describe the contingencies maintaining problem behavior at least as accurately as most adult observers.

Constructing the School–Home Note

After specifying the target behaviors, the consultant and other team members should begin "roughing out" the note. Many times the team can simply modify a note used previously. Sometimes teachers or guidance counselors will have used a particular type of school–home note in the past and recommend that it be modified to fit the current situation. Whenever possible, the consultant should accommodate these requests for using a familiar note, as long as doing so will not dilute the integrity of the procedure.

A number of features are important to include in the school–home note. The note should provide space for the child's name and the date. The consultant should attempt to make the note a convenient size—preferably about 5 in. × 8 in., or at least small enough that the child can place the note on his or her desk, yet large enough that it can be easily spotted. My colleagues and I recommend that colored paper be used with younger children so that the note can be easily seen amidst other papers.

As shown in Figure 4.3, Appendix 4.2, and the earlier figures depicting school–home notes, the note should specify the target behaviors and varying levels of performance for each behavior. The performance levels should be small enough that relatively small changes in behavior can be detected, yet global enough that the note does not provide an overwhelming amount of information. We find that the necessary level of detail concerning the target behavior varies across children and situations. When the child's behavior in a specific area is particularly problematic, then that behavior probably should

SCHOOL–HOME NOTE

Name __Matt_____   **Date** _____

SUBJECT__Reading_____

   Completed Classwork   YES SO-SO NO NA   Homework
                                              Assignment:
   Handed in Completed Homework YES SO-SO NO NA

Comments:

SUBJECT__Math_____

   Completed Classwork   YES SO-SO NO NA   Homework
                                              Assignment:
   Handed in Completed Homework YES SO-SO NO NA

Comments:

SUBJECT__Phonics_____

   Completed Classwork   YES SO-SO NO NA   Homework
                                              Assignment:
   Handed in Completed Homework YES SO-SO NO NA

Comments:

SUBJECT__Science/Social Studies___

   Completed Classwork   YES SO-SO NO NA   Homework
                                              Assignment:
   Handed in Completed Homework YES SO-SO NO NA

Comments:

SUBJECT__Spelling_____

   Completed Classwork   YES SO-SO NO NA   Homework
                                              Assignment:
   Handed in Completed Homework YES SO-SO NO NA

Comments:

FIGURE 4.3. School–home note for use with a child of elementary school age.

SCHOOL–HOME NOTE *(continued)*

Obeyed Classroom Rules (A.M.)   YES   SO-SO   NO
Obeyed Classroom Rules (P.M.)   YES   SO-SO   NO

Comments:

_____

Parent Comments:

_____

be assessed in a more fine-grained manner. For example, if a child's rate of work completion is his or her most serious problem and the child usually behaves in a cooperative manner during class, then work completion in each class subject should be broken down into smaller increments than other classroom behaviors. The note in Figure 4.3 illustrates this point: It is designed for a child whose academic work is the primary problem, so the child's adherence to classroom rules is evaluated only twice a day. More information is not always better and may in fact detract from the effectiveness of the school–home note. Too many data may result in the child's and other team members' being confused about the criteria for satisfactory performance. In addition, although it is important that performance criteria be operationalized, this level of specificity does not need to be evident on the actual note. For example, the criteria for "Behaved cooperatively in class" should be operationally defined, yet the note may only require the teacher to evaluate whether or not the behavior occurred.

The note should be uncluttered and appealing to the child, given his or her developmental status. For example, a young child may have a note with simple drawings or happy faces to reflect satisfactory performance. The team may enhance the appeal of the note by placing colorful stickers on the card when good behavior occurs. Older children usually prefer that their notes be simple and relatively small. Particularly for an older child or adolescent, the note should not include behavior descriptors that the child's classmates may see as condescending or immature.

As shown in Figure 4.3, it is very useful for the child or the teacher to have a place for writing down the homework assignment given in each class. For many of our clients, homework completion is inadequate and a frequent source of parent–child conflict. Our clients often fail to bring home the necessary materials for homework completion, deny that they have any homework, or avoid studying for tests until the last possible opportunity. These behaviors can be extremely frustrating for parents. When the child's homework assignments and information about upcoming tests are described on the note, parents are better informed, and problems can often be avoided.

Finally, notes should contain a place for teachers to comment about the child's behavior and to initial their evaluations. Teachers should use ink to reduce forgery attempts; parents should be wary about any erasures or changes in the note and should generally be aware that the child may be tempted to forge the teacher's evaluations or signature. Instances of forged notes should be mildly punished. For example, the child may be required to write an age-appropriate essay on why it is important to do well in school or on why it is important to tell the truth.

Teachers often appreciate getting feedback from parents about whether promised consequences were delivered, any comments about the previous day's evaluation, or questions about the child's assignments. We often ask teachers whether they would like to receive this information and include a space for parents to provide their comments on the school–home note. The child simply brings the completed note back to school the next day. Requiring the child to return the note with the parent's and teacher's comments from the previous day reduces the likelihood that the child will attempt to modify markings on the card. Figure 4.4 shows a completed school–home note with both teacher and parent comments. For the sake of brevity, only a portion of the note is shown.

Teachers' cooperation with the program can be enhanced when they are provided with information on how their evaluations are utilized and documentation that the parents have performed their agreed-upon responsibilities. This is particularly helpful in situations where parents and teachers have failed to communicate consistently, positively, or productively. An additional advantage to providing teachers with daily comments from parents is that the information often prompts the teachers to engage in positive interactions with the child about rewards, to remind the child of the consequences for good behavior, and to praise satisfactory performance.

NEGOTIATING BEHAVIOR CHANGE CONTRACTS

Specifying the Consequences for Classroom Behavior

Children's cooperation with a school–home note program is greatly affected by the rewards and encouragement they receive from their parents and teachers. Involving children in the selection of rewards

SCHOOL–HOME NOTE

Name ___Ashley_____ **Date** ___4/15_____

CLASS__Reading_____

    Followed instructions   Yes So-So No NA
    Completed classwork satisfactorily   Yes So-So No NA

    Homework/Test Grades   A B C D F NA

Comments:

CLASS__Math_____

    Followed instructions   Yes So-So No NA
    Completed classwork satisfactorily   Yes So-So No NA

    Homework/Test Grades   A B C D F NA

Comments:

CLASS__Phonics/Spelling_

    Followed instructions   Yes So-So No NA
    Completed classwork satisfactorily   Yes So-So No NA

    Homework/Test Grades   A B C D F NA

Comments:

Parent Comments:
    Consequences Provided Last Night:_Ashley watched TV for an hour and

    had 20 minutes of special time._

    Comments About Homework:_Ashley worked on her math facts._

    Other Comments:_Thanks for completing the note! I feel better able to

    help Ashley._

FIGURE 4.4. Abbreviated school–home note emphasizing parent comments.

can be exciting for them and communicates that their efforts at behavior change are appreciated. Many times, use of children's suggestions results in establishing more fair, accurate, and rewarding contingencies, and therefore increases the likelihood that behavior change will occur and be maintained over time.

In the clinical process whereby the program is developed and implemented, generating the contingencies for satisfactory performance usually occurs just prior to the first day of using the school–home note. Because the first week is typically reserved for baseline data collection, children earn rewards for simply obtaining the teacher's evaluations and bringing the completed notes home. In this way, the initial requirements for earning rewards are minimal, and the child is likely to meet them. Minimal initial requirements help insure that the program will begin on a positive note and provide parents and teachers with opportunities to practice praising good behavior. In addition, parent–child conflicts are often avoided when initial contingencies focus on increased privileges and minimal changes in behavior. When the child must meet a more stringent criterion to earn rewards, he or she will be in the habit of bringing the note home.

Generally, only the child, parents, and consultant are involved in negotiating privileges and sanctions. Occasionally, the parents may want to include other adults who control important rewards, such as an afternoon babysitter. If an adult is absent from the meeting but will be expected to provide consequences in a contingent manner, the consultant should obtain that person's consent to participate prior to determining the consequences. Teachers and other school personnel usually do not participate in this aspect of the program unless they will be providing additional consequences at school. They should, however, be provided with copies of the contract specifying the consequences for satisfactory and unsatisfactory behavior.

Prior to generating rewards, parents should be instructed to be positive, cooperative, and facilitative during the upcoming discussions with their child. They should be encouraged to compromise about privileges and attempt to make the school–home note program truly motivating and reinforcing for their child. For example, parents need to provide some rewards that children inconsistently or infrequently receive, so that children perceive parents as also putting forth some effort. My colleagues and I often tell parents that the program will be greatly enhanced by the degree to which they are able to be positive about their children's improvements and cooperation with the program (no matter how minimal), and that any negativism about their children or their involvement in the program should be avoided.

With older children or adolescents and their parents, we often provide some communication ground rules. A copy of these rules is presented in Table 4.3. As shown in the table, parents and their children are reminded to stay on the topic and to avoid interrupting and blaming one another. When clear expectations about communication are provided prior to any discussion of rewards, family conflict may be reduced or more easily dealt with when it does occur. Of course, the communication guidelines need to be tailored to the age and developmental status of the child.

The team members should be instructed to generate a list of daily and weekly rewards, as well as the conditions under which the consequences are provided. For example, the reward menu may state that the child can choose two daily rewards from the menu but that extra snacks are allowable only three times a week. Or the child may have the opportunity to earn two weekend privileges, but can only have a friend spend the night every other week. Table 4.4 lists activities that we have found are often rewarding to young elementary school children, older children, and adolescents.

The reward menu should include those that are normally available to the child regardless of his or her classroom behavior, and that the parent is comfortable both withholding when they are not earned and providing when deserved. For example, the child may routinely watch television upon returning home from school or eat a special snack at bedtime. These rewards are the type of daily activities that occur routinely and that parents are often willing to provide on a contingent basis. In establishing reward menus, parents should be encouraged to evaluate carefully whether they will feel guilty or resentful about withholding a specific privilege. For example, some parents may be unwilling to consider stories at bedtime a privilege, because they believe it is important to spend this time with their child regardless of his or her behavior. Other rewards may be viewed as too

TABLE 4.3. Communication Guidelines for Promoting Teacher–Family Problem Solving

Communication Ground Rules
1. Stick to the topic.
2. Avoid interrupting one another.
3. Avoid lecturing, criticizing, blaming.
4. Discuss goals and expectations ("I would like you to . . .").
5. Provide solutions to problems.
6. Use "I would like . . ." statements.
7. Avoid "You never . . .," "You always . . ." statements.
8. Do compromise.

TABLE 4.4. Daily and Weekly Rewards for Use with Children of Varying Ages

Daily	Weekly
Preschool and early elementary	
Late bedtime	Lunch at a fast-food restaurant
Twenty minutes with Mom or Dad	Having a friend over
	Small toy
Playing outside	Trip to park
10–25 cents	Friday night late bedtime
Snack	
Stories at bedtime	
Late elementary to junior high school	
Playing outside	Spending the night out or having a friend over
Computer games	
50 cents–$1	Going to mall/movie with parents and friend
25 cents for school snack	
TV	Wearing eyeshadow
	New T-shirt or small toy
Junior high to high school	
Use of the telephone	Going out Friday/Saturday night
$1–$3 (if money is not available in other ways)	Transportation to an activity
	Use of car
Not having to do the dishes	Later curfew
One hour of privacy after school	Going to the mall with a friend
	Money for clothes
No parental nagging after school	Double date once a month

time-consuming to provide on a regular basis, and therefore will be resented or inconsistently provided if included on the reward menu.

In many cases, the consultant, along with the team members, can brainstorm and suggest modifications in current activities so that a variety of rewards are generated. For example, parents may be unwilling to allow a child to stay up past his or her current bedtime of 8:30, and thus the child's request for a later bedtime is not an acceptable privilege. However, they may be very willing to change the child's standard weekday bedtime to 8:00, with the later bedtime thus becoming 8:30. In addition, they may consider an *extra* late Friday night bedtime of 10:00 appropriate.

Children may sometimes feel they are simply being "punished" for not doing better in school when normally available activities are made contingent on improved school performance. My colleagues and I offset this perception of punishment by including privileges in the reward menu that are generated by the children themselves. We enlist children in coming up with things that they would like to have but are not getting on a routine basis, and we encourage parents to strike some compromises to promote children's enthusiasm for the program. For example, children who normally are required to complete their homework before playing outside may feel that an important compromise has been reached if they are allowed to play outside for a period of time before beginning their homework. In this instance, parents may feel that an hour of outdoor play is a small price to pay for improved grades. We have found that providing children with a small amount of money to buy snacks or drinks at school is often a powerful incentive as well.

The enthusiasm of older children and adolescents can often be sparked by including privileges considered "grown-up." With children above the age of 10, a number of activities involving peers can serve as very powerful incentives. For example, older children may view riding their bikes to a neighborhood store or camping out in the back yard with friends as "grown-up" privileges that are only occasionally, if ever, provided by their parents. Adolescents often find it worth cooperating with a school–home note system in order to have extended use of the telephone, a later curfew, or independent shopping opportunities. The inclusion of "no parental nagging about school" or other types of reduced "invasions of privacy," such as "30 minutes of no questions upon returning home from school," also may be a powerful reward for the adolescent client. Of course, parents must feel comfortable about providing an older child or adolescent with opportunities for increased freedom from parental supervision. We strongly encourage parents, however, to maintain a spirit of compromise; we also emphasize that obtaining children's cooperation and maintaining their enthusiasm are important to the success of any contingency management program. In addition, systematically providing coveted privileges may reduce family arguments about whether a child or adolescent is "responsible," "old," or "good" enough to enjoy the freedom.

Although some authors suggest that punishment should not be included in a school–home note program, my colleagues and I believe that including some sanctions for unsatisfactory performance, in addition to rewards for good behavior, can enhance program effectiveness. For example, when children are not allowed to engage in their usual after-school activities (e.g., watching TV) because they did not earn the privilege, parents are perplexed about what to have the children do during this time period. Sometimes children do not appear particularly bothered by losing the privilege because so many other reinforcing activities are available to them. In these situations, we usually specify what the children will do when unable to experience their privileges. For example, a child may be required to write a short essay or copy some sentences about the importance of doing well in school. The essay should discuss the consequences of appropriate and inappropriate classroom behavior, and should focus on the particular behaviors that have resulted in the loss of privileges. Alternative negative consequences can include extra chores, copying homework assignments, or writing spelling words.

Parents should always specify sanctions for unsatisfactory performance in advance and should never add an aversive component to the program spontaneously and out of anger. For example, if children are to complete an extra chore instead of enjoying the privilege of playing outside or watching TV, they should be told in *advance* of the negative consequence for unsatisfactory behavior. Punishment should be provided in a calm manner and should only be recommended when the consultant is confident that the parents will not overdo the punishment. The consultant should strongly discourage the use of spanking or other physical punishment procedures. Thus, although some aversive consequences may be included in the program, parents should be encouraged to emphasize the use of rewards and praise as the primary tools for changing behavior. Guidelines for providing sanctions are presented in Table 4.5. (The use of two types

TABLE 4.5. Guidelines for Parents: Providing Sanctions for Unsatisfactory Behavior

1. Only deliver sanctions that are planned in advance, included in a contract, and fully expected by children. Children should have full knowledge of the sanction prior to beginning the contract.
2. Always provide a rationale whenever punishment is delivered.
3. Make the sanction relatively brief, relevant to the misbehavior, and constructive. Examples: an extra chore, additional practice at writing spelling words, recopying a failed test, writing a 150-word essay about the importance of not fighting.
4. Negotiate appropriate sanctions with your child.
5. Avoid using sanctions out of anger, frustration, or embarrassment. Sanctions are intended to instruct and increase the potency of incentives.
6. Deliver sanctions in a calm manner.
7. Do *not* use harsh, embarrassing, cruel, or physical sanctions or reprimands.
8. If you are *not* fully confident of your ability to deliver sanctions calmly, avoid their use. Instead, rely solely on reward-based approaches to improving behavior.

Note. Sanctions should not be recommended to parents with anger management problems or those who tend to be excessively negative with their children.

of negative consequences—response cost and overcorrection—is discussed further in Chapter 5.)

After the rewards and sanctions for satisfactory and unsatisfactory performance have been generated, my colleagues and I recommend that the contingencies be clearly spelled out in a contract. Figure 4.5 shows an example of a completed contract, including daily and weekly rewards. The contract specifies the conditions under which various rewards are provided, as well as what Timothy must do to earn the rewards. The contract also specifies a sanction for unsatisfactory behavior, which in this case is failing to bring the completed note home. Both the child and parents should sign the contract. A school–home note contract and record form that we have found useful are provided in Appendix 4.3.

With preschool children, a sticker or star chart and list of rewards often serve as an alternative to a contract. In this situation, the child earns a sticker or star for each instance of good performance. Performance criteria are read aloud to the child, and the child is asked to repeat the rules as well as what privileges will be earned. A parent handout on how to set up a star chart is provided in Appendix 4.4.

Negotiating Performance Goals

Generally, performance goals are established after the collection of at least 1 week's worth of baseline data. The activity involves reviewing the child's completed school–home notes and evaluating the quality of the feedback derived from using the procedure. If the note card provides relevant information about the child's behavior and does not need to be significantly modified, performance criteria can be based on the child's baseline performance.

Usually the consultant, parents, and teachers participate in establishing performance criteria. Children should be encouraged to participate and to express their opinions about performance goals in a manner commensurate with their age and abilities. Although children's abilities to offer accurate accounts of their behavior will vary considerably, their opinions should be prompted, and the situation should be used as an opportunity to begin teaching self-evaluation skills.

In establishing performance criteria, we often use the problem-solving steps shown in Table 4.6 as a communication guide. The problem-solving steps are adapted from material presented in Robin and Foster (1989). Use of this model is particularly helpful with older children and adolescents, who tend to be defensive and occasionally resistant to the idea of using a school–home note program.

SCHOOL–HOME NOTE CONTRACT RECORD

Name Timothy   **Date** 11/1-11/5

A good note is: When Timothy completes at least 75% of his classwork correctly in 5 of 7 subjects.

If a good note is earned: Timothy plays outside, earns 25 cents, and gets a special snack.

If a good note is not earned: Timothy must copy spelling words 10 times or do an extra chore (Mom or Dad chooses).

If a note is forgotten: Timothy must copy a paragraph on the importance of doing schoolwork and complete an extra chore.

If 4/5 good notes are brought home by the end of the week: Timothy gets lunch out and a special activity with Dad.

If fewer than 3 good notes are brought home: Timothy does not receive rewards.

DAILY RECORD OF NOTES	CONSEQUENCES PROVIDED
Monday: 75% in 5/7	Received rewards (25 cents)
Tuesday: 75% in 6/7	Received rewards
Wednesday: 75% in 6/7	Received rewards
Thursday: 75% in 4/7	No rewards, mopped kitchen
Friday: 75% in 5/7	Extra 25 cents because couldn't play
Weekly: 4/5 good days!	Fishing w/Dad; lunch at McDonald's

FIGURE 4.5. Timothy's completed contract and summary of the week's performance. The form used here was developed by Ginger K. Kendell, Louisiana State University, 1989. Used by permission.

Beginning with "Defining the problem," the consultant should encourage the team members to summarize the child's school–home note evaluations obtained during the previous week. Their statements should attempt to objectively describe (1) levels of performance for various target behaviors; (2) variations in performance levels across situations; and (3) factors believed to be associated with satisfactory

TABLE 4.6. Problem-Solving Steps for Use in Negotiating Solutions to Conflicts, with Emphasis on Academic and Classroom Behavior

<u>Problem-Solving as a Negotiation Tool</u>

1. *Set the stage*
   A. Choose a problem to discuss.
   B. Choose a time and place to discuss the problem.
   C. Review steps to problem solving.
   D. Review Communication Ground Rules.

2. *Define the problem*
   A. Each person states what words or actions are problematic.
   B. Stick to the facts and the topic.
   C. Each person is likely to present a different description of the problem; avoid criticizing one another's definitions.

3. *Generate solutions*
   A. Think up and record as many solutions to the problem as you can (6–10).
   B. Team members should take turns offering solutions.
   C. Follow the rules for brainstorming: Do not judge solutions.
   D. Record solutions on a worksheet.
   E. Solutions can include specific modifications in the classroom or homework routines, ways of improving performance, and incentives.

4. *Evaluate solutions: Decision making*
   A. Evaluate the long-term and short-term, positive and negative consequences of each solution.
   B. Each team member should rate how much he or she likes each solution.
   C. Add additional solutions.
   D. Compromise and include incentives for using the solutions.
   E. Remember to use the Communication Ground Rules.
   F. Attempt to come up with specific behavior goals and incentives for goal achievement.

5. *Plan implementation*
   A. Record chosen solution on a contract.
   B. Discuss obstacles to using the solutions and achieving expected performance.

6. *Evaluate performance*
   A. Monitor contract fulfillment daily.

Note. Adapted from *Negotiating Parent–Adolescent Conflict: A Behavioral Family Systems Approach* by A. L. Robin and S. L. Foster, 1989 (pp. 193–194). New York: Guilford Press. Copyright 1989 by The Guilford Press. Adapted by permission.

and unsatisfactory behavior (e.g., difficult material, seating arrangement for a particular class). Team members should be reminded to emphasize positive aspects of behavior, rather than focusing only on negative behavior such as the child's failures. When appropriate, the child can be encouraged to comment on the feedback as well. Teachers should also be asked whether this baseline performance seems representative of the child's general performance. As recommended in the problem-solving guide, all team members should be encouraged to provide a description of the problem and their goals for problem solving. Disagreements about the problem and why problem behaviors occur are common and need not be resolved (Robin & Foster, 1984).

My colleagues and I suggest that the process of defining the problem be assertively directed by the consultant. The consultant should move the discussion forward and offer his or her opinions throughout the process. We do not consider problem-solving skills acquisition to be a primary objective of setting up a school–home note program. Although use of the problem-solving model may serve therapeutic functions, it is mainly recommended as a method of guiding communication. When appropriate, team members should be reminded of the communication ground rules and encouraged to practice positive communication behavior. Emphasis on communication and the child's involvement in problem solving must, of course, be appropriate for the situation and the child's developmental status.

After defining the problems reflected in the school–home notes completed the previous week, team members should begin "Generating solutions" and establish performance goals for the next week. During this problem-solving phase, the team members should list as many solutions as possible and avoid evaluating solutions until later. Both our own experience and research suggest that generating many solutions increases the likelihood that an effective solution will be obtained.

Although rewards for goal achievement will always be a component of the school–home note program, additional problem solutions are sometimes suggested. Modifications in the classroom routine and other stimulus control interventions should always be considered as possible ways of enhancing the effectiveness of school–home notes. For example, a teacher may suggest that the child be moved to a seat in the front of the classroom to reduce the opportunity to talk to classmates, or may recommend that more frequent monitoring of the child's independent classwork take place. The child may suggest methods of increasing his or her organization and "remembering" skills, in order to improve the consistency with which he or she brings home materials and books necessary for completing homework. The parents may suggest ways of establishing a more effective after-school routine so that homework is supervised more closely.

In establishing performance criteria, the teachers, parents, and, when appropriate, the child should discuss the level of improvement that the child can be expected to make in a short period of time. We recommend that only small changes in behavior be expected in the beginning. It is easier to adjust the criteria upward as children achieve performance goals than it is to lower stringent standards after children have failed to meet them. Lowering standards may communicate to children that failure will result in decreased expectations and easier access to rewards; obviously, this is not the message that parents wish to communicate.

In general, my colleagues and I suggest that the performance criteria represent about a 20–30% improvement over baseline performance, although this amount will vary, depending on the specific target behaviors and the child's pretreatment performance. We suggest requiring improved performance across most time periods or classes in which the child's baseline performance is not acceptable. For example, if the child completes only about 30% of his or her classwork assignments correctly, the goal may be to increase this rate to 50% in most of the child's classes (e.g., five of seven), as opposed to requiring a larger improvement in fewer classes (e.g., 70% in three of seven classes).

With many children, a primary goal is to increase the consistency with which they perform required work. These children sometimes complete their work satisfactorily and at other times do not. We believe that consistent work performance is best accomplished by requiring small amounts of improvement across many opportunities, rather than relatively large changes in a small number of situations. To help circumvent the problem of children only doing a "little bit better" because they earn rewards for small changes, we sometimes maintain a two-level incentive system. The system requires only small changes in behavior across most situations, but specifies that an important "bonus" incentive should be provided when the child's performance substantially exceeds the minimal criteria.

The next problem-solving step is "Evaluating solutions" to come up with the optimal problem-solving approach. This phase usually involves reviewing the list of solutions; having each team member evaluate how well he or she believes the solution would work to solve or partially solve the problem; and then pooling solutions to come up with the "best" method, given the evaluations. We suggest that the consultant take a fairly directive role in this process, guiding the members to combine solutions that represent a compromise among the individuals involved. Frequently, it is evident to the consultant that solutions can be combined in ways that are likely to produce the best overall solution. For example, the consultant may be able to come up with compromises overlooked by team members. We recommend that the consultant provide these solutions and guide the team to engage in focused, positive discussions.

As in other aspects of setting up a school–home note program, a child's role in the program should increase with age. In general, preschoolers may be asked for their opinions, but the major portion of their input will be to assist with generating rewards for good behavior. Adolescents should have a much greater role in generating solutions and formulating program goals and contingencies.

The reward–punishment portion of the contingency is usually already in place before performance criteria are established. However, the consultant should review how well the incentives have worked and whether the consequences have been provided consistently. We suggest that the consultant carefully ascertain whether the child perceives the reinforcers as "worth" the expected behavior change, and if not, how the rewards might be enhanced to increase their potency. Small changes in the reward menu often significantly increase children's productive involvement in the school–home note program.

We recommend that the consultant briefly interview an older child or adolescent separately from the adult team members when reviewing the fairness and effectiveness of instituted contracts. This time gives the child an opportunity for freer discussion of the school–home note and the rewards associated with improved performance; as such, it promotes the child's cooperation with the program.

After determining the optimal combination of solutions to the child's problems, the consultant and team members should describe the specific behaviors, performance goals, and rewards for goal achievement in a new contract. The consultant should aid the team in specifying the precise behaviors the child, parents, and teachers will perform to fulfill the contract, including exactly how rewards and sanctions will be provided. All areas of ambiguity should be clarified, and clarifications should be written into the contract as discussed previously. We usually recommend that the contract remain in effect for at least 1–2 weeks, to allow the procedure time to work before being changed or discontinued.

IMPLEMENTING THE PROGRAM

Initiating Treatment

After careful selection of target behaviors, performance goals, and consequences for goal achievement, the actual administration of the school–home note program sometimes seems relatively easy. However, several components of the program should be reviewed before the procedure is actually begun, and then should be monitored throughout the program. For example, the consultant must insure that the school–home note program is administered in a positive and fair way, so that children feel good about working toward improving their classroom behavior.

To implement the school–home note program successfully, the consultant should discuss the role each team member plays in administering the procedure. This presentation should describe (1) who is responsible for completing the note; (2) how active the child should be in obtaining the evaluations; (3) when and how parents and teachers will praise satisfactory performance and reprimand or punish unsatisfactory performance; (4) how the procedure will be integrated into the classroom and home routines; and (5) what, if any, additional interventions will be used to augment the effectiveness of the program.

With regard to delineating responsibilities, my colleagues and I generally recommend that the teacher(s) be responsible for completing the note and giving the note to the child to bring home. With a younger child, the teacher should have blank notes on hand for completion, although parents generally are responsible for providing the copies. An older child or an adolescent usually is responsible for giving a blank note to the teacher at the beginning of the day and picking up the note from the teacher at the end of the day or class period. Parents are responsible for providing privileges in a contingent manner and making sure homework is completed correctly and on time.

In the beginning, a child may forget to ask the teacher to complete the note or to pick the note up from the teacher. We suggest taking a positive approach to increasing a child's responsibility in the program, rather than viewing instances of forgetfulness as yet another example of the student's laziness, disinterest, or disorganization. Teachers should be encouraged to praise children when "remembering" occurs and to provide neutral prompts when children forget, particularly during early phases of the program. In addition, children should not receive their privileges if they fail to bring their notes home. However, if problems with "forgetfulness" persist, the contract can be upgraded to specify consequences for obtaining the completed note without teacher prompting.

When a school–home note program is first being implemented, and whenever performance criteria are changed, teachers and parents should remind children of the standards for earning privileges before the day begins. For example, Timothy's teacher may say, "Timothy, today you will earn your rewards if you complete 80% of your assignments correctly. You can do less well on one assignment and still receive your rewards. Yesterday you achieved your goal. Let's see if we can have another really good day."

Teachers and parents can increase children's awareness of performance goals and rewards for goal achievement by requiring them to recite the contingencies. For example, after stating the rules for earning good ratings, Timothy's teacher may say, "OK, tell me what you have to do to get a 'yes' on your note." After Timothy answers correctly, the teacher asks, "What happens if you earn nine 'yes' marks?" As children become familiar with their goals, they may be required to state the criteria without having the information provided first. For example, after Timothy has been reminded of his performance standards on one or two occasions, his teacher may ask, "Timothy, what do you have to do to earn your rewards for good behavior?", rather than simply telling Timothy the information.

By encouraging children to state the rules for good behavior, teachers and parents may increase the salience of the contingencies and children's use of self-instructions for managing behavior. It is our general belief that through shaping children's ability to specify the consequences for satisfactory and unsatisfactory performance, adults promote self-managed behavior. My colleagues and I believe that it is through experiencing explicitly stated overt contingencies that children's covert use of self-instruction, self-evaluation, and self-reinforcement is developed. These skills are necessary for a child to maintain adequate progress after the school–home note program is faded out later.

In a similar vein, we recommend that teachers provide children with frequent feedback about their behavior throughout the day and encourage children to evaluate how well they are behaving in relation to their goals. Ideally, teachers should inform children of their ratings after each evaluation interval. For example, if a child is evaluated after each class period, the teacher should attempt to provide the child with the ratings after each class. We find that feedback to the child can be increased when the school–home note is placed on the child's desk and the teacher goes to the child's desk to complete the card. Although some teachers find this practice inconvenient, others do not believe it creates much additional work: They simply check over the child's work, complete the note, and provide feedback during a single trip to the child's desk.

As children become familiar with their performance criteria, we recommend that teachers and parents prompt children to evaluate their own behavior. For example, a child who is rewarded for completing a specific amount of classwork can be asked whether he or she did or did not achieve the goal for a given class period. A child who earns privileges based on operationally defined criteria of being prepared for class, not bothering other students, and using class time well can be asked to judge the degree to which he or she was successful in each area. Of course, prompting children's self-evaluations can only be done as time permits, but we do suggest that teachers attempt to do this at least once or twice a day.

We have found that some younger children or children with significant learning or cognitive deficits are unable to assess whether they were successful at achieving their goals. Sometimes these children are uncertain as to whether they behaved in a satisfactory manner even when teachers and parents try to give concrete, specific feedback. In part, this problem can be avoided by constructing a school–home note that is very simple and includes only one or two target behaviors. However, we have found that children who have difficulty interpreting the information on the note can benefit from the use of stickers placed beside each evaluation when they have performed satisfactorily. For example, I used a school–home note program with a very inattentive, mildly retarded child (Keith) who also had numerous learning and behavior problems. Two of my primary goals were (1) to increase Keith's completion of academic work and (2) to reduce his disruptive behavior, including talking without permission. Keith attended a special school for learning-disabled students and changed classes for his various academic subjects. An abbreviated version of Keith's school–home note is shown in Figure 4.6. As shown in the figure, each of his teachers completed the note based on Keith's behavior in his or her class. As Keith often appeared to misunderstand his teachers' comments and evaluations, I asked each instructor to provide Keith with a sticker if he behaved in a satisfactory manner in class. I defined satisfactory performance as receiving no more than one "no" in a single academic subject. Keith was rewarded at home for receiving at least five of seven stickers that day. Requiring the teachers to provide stickers not only made the evaluation criteria and contingencies of reinforcement more salient, but also created opportunities for more immediate, positive feedback from the teacher. I believe that use of the stickers served some reinforcing

SCHOOL–HOME NOTE

Name___Keith_____   **Date** ____2/25_____

SUBJECT___Math_____

Sticker

Brought Materials   (YES)   SO-SO   NO
Completed Classwork   YES   (SO-SO)   NO   ★
Kept Hands to Self   YES   SO-SO   (NO)

Comments: Keith worked pretty well but he frequently poked the boy in front of him.

SUBJECT___Reading_____

Sticker

Brought Materials   (YES)   SO-SO   NO
Completed Classwork   (YES)   SO-SO   NO   ★
Kept Hands to Self   (YES)   SO-SO   NO

Comments: Did well.

SUBJECT___Spelling_____

Sticker

Brought Materials   (YES)   SO-SO   NO
Completed Classwork   YES   (SO-SO)   NO   ★
Kept Hands to Self   YES   (SO-SO)   NO

Comments:

SUBJECT___English_____

Sticker

Brought Materials   YES   SO-SO   (NO)
Completed Classwork   YES   SO-SO   (NO)
Kept Hands to Self   YES   (SO-SO)   NO

Comments: Did not have notebook.

SUBJECT___Social Values___

Sticker

Brought Materials   (YES)   SO-SO   NO
Completed Classwork   (YES)   SO-SO   NO   ★
Kept Hands to Self   (YES)   SO-SO   NO

Comments: Great day!

FIGURE 4.6. Keith's school–home note.

functions and prompted teachers to praise Keith more frequently for behaving in a satisfactory manner. Keith reported enjoying the stickers and looked forward to picking them out at the consultant's office.

Another important way for teachers to increase children's awareness of their progress toward goal achievement is to praise them frequently for exhibiting appropriate behavior. My colleagues and I generally find that teachers' use of praise and encouragement throughout the day is integral to children's success in the program. Without adequate encouragement and feedback, the delay in reinforcement that naturally accompanies the school–home note may be too lengthy to alter behavior.

Although use of a school–home note reduces some of teachers' concerns about providing "special" treatment to a single child, some teachers are opposed to "catching the child being good" on a frequent basis. They may feel (as do some parents) that children should not be praised excessively for performing routine behaviors. They may believe that giving one child extra attention through praise and other forms of reinforcement may cause classmates to misbehave to receive equivalent consequences. These and other concerns about contingent reinforcement voiced by teachers should be addressed. One rationale we frequently provide to teachers is that research suggests that praising one child for engaging in appropriate behavior often serves to prompt other students to engage in similar behavior. For example, we discuss how praise may be used as a method of teaching children how and when to engage in appropriate behavior. Table 4.7 provides a list of the behaviors to recommend to parents and teachers for effectively praising children.

It is very important that parents spend time reviewing and discussing the completed note each day. We suggest that parents review teachers' comments in the order in which they were written, so that an overview of the child's behavior throughout the day is presented. For example, if the child's first class is math, then ratings of behavior exhibited during math should be reviewed first. At times, it may be difficult for parents to go patiently through the teachers' evaluations when a particularly poor evaluation was given. However, by systematically reviewing the teachers' comments in a neutral manner, parents minimize the temptation to overreact and focus excessively on negative comments. Predictable, relatively calm parental responses, in turn, can result in improved communication between parents and children.

Parents should encourage children to comment on the ratings and to evaluate their own behavior as the completed note is reviewed. Again, this can help children understand exactly what they must do to

TABLE 4.7. Recommended Procedures for Praising Children in an Instructive, Warm Manner

---

Giving Positive Attention

1. *Make praise specific.*

   Tell the child *exactly* what he or she did that was positive. Praise immediately following the behavior.

   Example: "Jill, you completed your math very quickly and you got all but two answers correct. I'm very pleased."

2. *Make praise enjoyable.*

   Praise in an enthusiastic, sincere manner. Children are very skilled at detecting anger and frustration. Insincere praise may only hurt rather than help.

3. *Praise frequently.*

   Although the need to reprimand children will never be eliminated, praise should occur far more frequently than corrections. One way to use praise to improve classroom behavior is to praise the well-behaved child in a specific manner. The praise often serves to remind the misbehaving child of the household or classroom rules.

4. *Make praise contingent.*

   Only praise when the child is behaving in a positive manner. Avoid using praise and compliments as methods of coaxing good behavior from children who are misbehaving.

5. *Use praise to instruct.*

   Use praise to teach children *how* to behave by acknowledging components of a newly acquired skill.

   Example: A child beginning to learn two-digit addition should be praised in a specific manner for the problems completed correctly.

6. *Pair praise with additional incentives.*

   It is useful to accompany praise with a more tangible acknowledgment. For example, teachers may include an added incentive for a very good school–home note. Initial efforts at promoting a new behavior should include frequent rewards accompanied with praise.

7. *Carry out promised consequences.*

   Parent and teacher praise will only be meaningful if consequences are provided when promised. Avoid promising a reward that is uncomfortable or inconvenient to give.

8. *Give positive attention right away.*

   Give the child positive attention *while* good behavior is happening or *right after* a good behavior.

---

earn satisfactory evaluations; it also provides opportunities for parents to teach their children problem-solving skills. For example, when reviewing comments about inappropriate behavior, parents can ask their children how they may have handled the situation differently.

Like teachers' feedback, the feedback parents provide to children should be as positive as possible. The consultant should emphasize the importance of parents' shaping appropriate behavior through the use of frequent praise. Parents also should be instructed to praise children by describing the specific, appropriate behaviors exhibited. In this way, parents use praise as a tool for teaching their children how to behave. For example, Timothy's parents may praise him when he brings home a good note by saying, "Timothy, you did so well today. You completed 80% of your classwork in reading, spelling, English, math, and science. That is really terrific. You also behaved in a cooperative way in almost all subjects."

We find that parents often are uncomfortable or unskilled at praising children in an enthusiastic, specific way. Thus, it is often necessary for the consultant to provide a good deal of instruction and examples in the use of praise in order for parents to carry out a school–home note program effectively. We frequently model and role-play methods for praising children in a specific and sincere manner with parents and teachers. Table 4.7 is applicable to both parents and teachers.

The consultant should carefully monitor whether parents and teachers provide promised consequences in a fair, consistent, and positive manner. We suggest that a method of monitoring contract adherence be developed to increase parents' awareness of the importance of following through with the agreed-upon rewards. For example, the parent can list whether rewards are earned and given on a daily basis on a monitoring form or on the school–home note. Parents' monitoring of their own behavior also may serve to increase program compliance and provides a source of data for review by the consultant during follow-up sessions.

Parents may encounter numerous obstacles that limit their compliance with the contract. Sometimes, compliance is diminished due to decreased availability of the reward (e.g., the child could not play outside because of the weather) or inability of a parent to provide the consequence (e.g., the father worked late). Although problems with contract adherence are somewhat common, and many parents may make spontaneous changes in the contract to carry out the "spirit" of the agreement, parents should be advised to follow through with their commitments. Sometimes, even minor changes in rewards are viewed by children as a sign of "bad faith," resulting in diminished motivation to perform satisfactorily at school. Older children or adolescents occasionally view apparently insignificant contract changes as yet another example of their parents failure to take them seriously and appreciate their perspective. This type of resentment early in a school–home note program may result in an adolescent's refusing to cooperate with treatment and displaying a variety of nonfacilitative behaviors.

Given the potential problems that may arise if the contract is changed, parents should be advised to avoid making changes and to contact the consultant if problems arise in adhering to the contingency. During these discussions, which we have found often take place on the telephone, the consultant should carefully review with the parent the problems and the ways in which these were handled. The child's opinions about modifying the contract should be solicited by the parent and, when necessary, the consultant. In this way, both the child and the parent view contractual modifications as important. The consultant is also given an opportunity to direct the family to make changes considered acceptable by both parent and child. When changes are made in the contract, the parent or consultant should contact the child's teachers and inform them of the changes. If the changes are likely to affect the child's behavior at school or the teacher's involvement in the school–home note program, the teachers should be given an opportunity to discuss the suggested changes.

Evaluating Program Effectiveness

In many ways, program evaluation begins the first day of using the school–home note program. My colleagues and I view evaluation as integral to the day-to-day mechanics of competently administering the program. When treatment outcome is evaluated in an ongoing manner, the consultant's decisions to change performance criteria or the school–home note are based on data rather than subjective accounts.

Although the consultant has a major role in setting up and supervising program evaluation, the system should allow teachers, parents, and students to monitor program success on a day-by-day basis. For example, parental use of a star chart may serve as a method of monitoring how often a young child has achieved his or her goals over a month-long period. An older child may want to monitor achievement of daily goals using a graphing procedure and colored markers.

A school–home note program may be ineffective due to a variety of classroom, teacher, parent, or child variables. Table 4.8 shows a

TABLE 4.8. Checklist of Variables That Influence the Effectiveness of a School-Home Note Program

School-Home Note Program Checklist

Target behaviors

   1. ____ Target behaviors are defined in a specific manner.

   2. ____ Target behaviors occur frequently and are potentially sensitive to change.

   3. ____ The behaviors are judged as important by the teacher, parents, and student.

   4. ____ Target behavior definitions are understood by the parents, teacher, and student.

   5. ____ Target behaviors are easy for the teacher to monitor.

   6. ____ Target behaviors are worded positively.

   7. ____ Target behaviors are evaluated by the teacher in all relevant situations.

Evaluation criteria and performance goals

   1. ____ The evaluation anchors (e.g., happy vs. sad face) are well defined.

   2. ____ The parent, teacher, and student understand what behaviors warrant positive versus negative evaluations.

   3. ____ The child clearly understands what must be done to earn rewards.

   4. ____ The parent, teacher, and student agree that the required level of performance is fair and within the student's current ability to achieve.

   5. ____ Improvements in the student's performance result in improved global evaluations by parents and teacher.

The note

   1. ____ The actual school–home note is uncluttered, organized, and easy to complete.

   2. ____ The note is pleasing to the child and developmentally appropriate with regard to wording and performance criteria.

   3. ____ Data derived from the note are easy to summarize.

Administration

   1. ____ Parent, teacher, and student responsibilities are clear to all involved (e.g., it is understood who provides the blank note daily).

   2. ____ Each teacher completes the note daily and provides meaningful comments to the student and parent.

   3. ____ The note is minimally intrusive for the student and teacher.

   4. ____ The child is not ridiculed or excessively questioned by other students about the note.

   5. ____ Each teacher completes the note in a friendly, facilitative manner and avoids making hostile, embarrassing, or excessively critical statements to the child.

   6. ____ Parents provide feedback to the teacher about home consequences and ask questions when they arise.

   7. ____ Both the parents and teacher use the note as a communication tool rather than a weapon, and take time to acknowledge improvement and each other's problem-solving efforts.

(cont.)

TABLE 4.8. *(continued)*

8. _____ The note is used for at least a few weeks after behavior is quite acceptable and then faded systematically (or reintroduced if performance diminishes).

Feedback and consequences

1. _____ The target behavior goals and consequences for goal achievement are clear and written in a contract.
2. _____ The child earns both daily and weekly rewards.
3. _____ The child participates in generating the rewards for goal achievement.
4. _____ Rewards are important and *truly* rewarding to the child.
5. _____ Teacher provides feedback about performance and goal achievement at regular intervals throughout the day.
6. _____ Parents review the teacher's comments daily and promote improved performance through problem-solving with the child.
7. _____ Parents and teacher praise the child for goal achievement.

checklist of variables that may diminish the effectiveness of a school–home note system, produce conflict between parents and teachers, or decrease the social validity of the treatment program. For example, parents and teachers may not be providing adequate incentives for performance, given the salience of peer reinforcement for disruptive behavior. The target child may need to develop the skills necessary to complete the required work. Other common problems include disagreement among team members regarding target behavior definitions; unrealistic work goals; inadequate monitoring of the child's behavior; and insufficient feedback to the child regarding goal achievement. We suggest that the list shown in Table 4.8 be carefully reviewed with the team when assessing the causes for a lack of program effectiveness. The list also is helpful as a trouble-shooting guide for use prior to beginning the program.

Normally, the consultant meets with team members after giving the school–home note program sufficient time to begin working. My colleagues and I have found that a 1- to 2-week period of using the program is usually reasonable. Such a period allows the consultant to begin to evaluate program adherence and effectiveness, as well as to discuss problems and misunderstandings before they get out of hand. Although it is ideal to conduct a meeting with the teachers, parents, and child, this is sometimes impractical. Often, the consultant can talk separately with the parents and teacher to assess quickly whether the program is being implemented properly and to address minor problems. The meeting generally includes only the parents and child, although the consultant should have a good understanding of the teachers' opinions about the program and any recommendations for changing performance criteria.

If a teacher is dissatisfied with the program or would like many changes, an effort should be made to conduct a team meeting. For example, the child's teachers may feel that performance standards should be raised in some subjects but not others. They may believe that the parents are not receiving sufficient information or that the notes should be modified to target different behaviors.

Perhaps one of the biggest obstacles to effective use of a school–home note program is the temptation to alter or discontinue the program without ample opportunity to assess effectiveness. The consultant must determine carefully whether changes suggested by team members do in fact seem appropriate and beneficial. Often, the team members simply require more time to incorporate the procedure into their routines, and the child needs to learn that the contract will be strictly enforced. For example, we have experienced several cases in which a teacher or parent was ready to give up on the program because it did not seem to be working adequately. Two types of problems have often occurred: In some cases, there was a "honeymoon" effect, in which the program produced satisfactory behavior change during the first few days and then performance deteriorated; in other instances, the child's behavior did not substantially change or seemed to get worse than when treatment was first initiated. We sometimes recommend changes in the reward program or the administration of the procedure when the program does not work adequately. However, it is our experience that tenacious administration of the program in the absence of immediate behavior change eventually results in improved behavior in most cases.

Parents' and teachers' discouragement and frustration about program effectiveness must be addressed sensitively by the consultant. We often discuss the fact that a child's behavior problems have developed over a period of time and that he or she should be given ample time to "unlearn" bad habits and to acquire new skills. We remind team members that the program serves as a feedback system and that greater communication between parents and teachers is also a beneficial outcome. Finally, we discuss our experience with similar situations and describe the probable eventual outcomes.

Although the consultant should encourage parents and teachers to give the program a chance to work, he or she should also reassure them that an ineffective program will not be continued indefinitely. The consultant should communicate that he or she will attempt in an effortful and comprehensive manner to identify and correct problems interfering with program success. The consultant should also avoid creating the impression that a school-home note system *always* works or is *always* superior to other interventions.

As suggested earlier, my colleagues and I recommend that the consultant, along with the parents and child, develop a method of summarizing the information presented in the school-home note program. At the most basic level, the system should clearly indicate whether or not the child achieved criterion on a daily basis. Should it seem appropriate or helpful to provide feedback, the evaluation procedure can also summarize the percentage of intervals in which each of the target behaviors was or was not exhibited. For example, the consultant and team member may wish to know the percentage of the student's homework assignments that were handed in on time or the percentage of classes in which the child behaved cooperatively without talking out of turn.

We suggest that only the information needed to improve behavior be summarized formally. We do, however, strongly recommend that all sources of data be evaluated daily by the parent and child. For example, Timothy's performance graph may only identify the percentage of classes in which he performed satisfactorily. However, Timothy and his parents should review his performance in all areas nightly.

When specific target behaviors are performed inconsistently and/or appear to require additional focus to produce optimal behavior change, it is helpful to include these behaviors in a formal evaluation system. For example, if a child frequently talks without permission, as in Keith's case (see Figure 4.6), then this behavior may be summarized on a graph along with a record of the child's overall performance that day. The special emphasis on specific goals communicates to children that the target behavior is especially important to perform.

It is important to examine the social validity of the treatment when making judgments about program effectiveness. As discussed previously, social validity is concerned with consumers' opinions about the importance of treatment goals, procedures, and outcomes. If the treatment procedure is judged as unacceptable for whatever reason, team members will be unlikely to use the treatment with integrity or at all. For example, we have dealt with a number of situations in which the program apparently was working, but teachers or parents abruptly terminated its use.

The consultant should consider several aspects of social validity when evaluating treatment effectiveness. The consultant should determine whether improvements in the target behaviors are viewed as sufficiently important from the teacher's and parents' perspectives.

For example, we encountered one case in which a child almost always received very good marks from his teachers, but the teachers continued to complain about his behavior. In this situation, the target behaviors listed in the note did not adequately represent the disruptive behaviors considered problematic by the student's teachers. Thus, the treatment *goals* were inadequate for the consumers to judge the procedure as socially valid.

Sometimes parents and teachers may disagree about the significance of treatment outcome. For example, one party may feel that the child's behavior is improved, but the other still perceives the behavior as unacceptable. For a third-grade student, Owen, I used a school–home note program that focused on decreasing the boy's talking without permission. During baseline Owen talked without permission about 10 times a day. He engaged in numerous attention-seeking behaviors, such as making noises and blurting out silly, immature comments. The school–home note required him to cross out a number each time he was corrected. Owen earned rewards for minimal point loss. The teacher noted that, with treatment, Owen talked without permission about twice a day. In spite of this improvement, he received a D for his weekly conduct grade because he was corrected 10 times during the course of the week. In this case, the teacher recognized Owen's improvements but did not view the amount of change as adequate for a passing conduct grade.

Two issues surfaced when I discussed the situation with Owen's teacher. First, it appeared that the teacher's expectations became more stringent when the school–home note program was initiated; she began to expect more as the child's behavior improved during the week. Second, she was a particularly strict teacher who had fairly rigid standards of appropriate classroom behavior. Although the child's mother and the consultant viewed the child's behavior improvements as quite satisfactory, the teacher did not. In part, I responded by observing Owen in the classroom and comparing his behavior to that of other classmates.

Regardless of their initial willingness to use a school–home note program, parents and teachers sometimes dislike the procedure once they begin using it. They may feel that it is too much work, for example. Although dissatisfied team members may bring up their reservations spontaneously, more often than not attitudes about the program will be more passively communicated through inconsistent administration of the procedure. Thus, we have found that it is important to encourage parents and teachers to discuss any negative side effects or negative opinions about the treatment whenever they arise. Unless team members are given an "out" such as this, they may passively resist cooperating, and thus a potentially effective intervention may fail.

A school–home note program may have a number of negative side effects. Most of these are occasionally seen with any reinforcement-based program. Because the presence of negative side effects can greatly affect parents', teacher's and children's cooperation with the school–home note program, the consultant should assess them carefully. Many side effects can be easily addressed by modifying the daily report procedure in minor ways.

Common side effects that the consultant may inquire about directly include the following:

1. Teachers and parents may feel uncomfortable about giving the target child a disproportionate amount of time and attention, compared to other students or the child's siblings. They may complain that the other children are misbehaving more often in order to receive privileges.

2. Parents may report that the system is no longer working because the child does not seem interested in the rewards.

3. Teachers and parents may begin to complain that administration of the note is too time-consuming or disruptive. This may occur after a "honeymoon" period in which the treatment has been quite effective; the team members may have forgotten how difficult the child was to manage before beginning the note program.

4. The child may be questioned or teased about the note by classmates, or he or she may simply feel self-conscious about using the note and want to discontinue the procedure.

5. Either the parent or teacher may be administering the note in a negative manner and using punishment to bring about behavior change.

Fading the School–Home Note Program

After a period of consistent, satisfactory behavior, school–home note programs should be faded and eventually eliminated. My colleagues and I suggest that initial fading efforts be aimed at reducing the *amount* of feedback rather than *frequency* of feedback. That is, parents and teachers should provide less detailed feedback on a daily basis (e.g., overall rates of work completion for an entire school day), rather than reducing how often a detailed, comprehensive note is employed. For example, Timothy's school–home note can be modified so that the teacher evaluates whether Timothy has generally completed his classwork and behaved satisfactorily in the morning and afternoon. This feedback provides a more global indication of his behavior for two lengthy intervals on a daily basis. Over time, the teacher can provide even less feedback, so that Timothy is evaluated at the end of the school day only. Later, these daily evaluations can be sent home to the parents at the end of the week; teachers often provide this delayed, weekly feedback as a typical part of the classroom routine. Thus, school–home notes can be faded to the point where parents are provided weekly feedback based on daily, relatively global evaluations of behavior. Although we have encountered situations in which virtually all feedback to parents was eliminated, common sense would suggest that some regular feedback to parents should be maintained, particularly with younger children.

With older children and adolescents, the teacher's evaluations can be gradually replaced with self-evaluations. For example, students may be asked to monitor whether they have completed their classwork or turned in their homework. Initially, these evaluations can be obtained along with teacher evaluations and later compared to assess student accuracy. As the student demonstrates the ability to monitor his or her behavior accurately, teacher evaluations can be obtained less frequently. For example, after a period of using a teacher-administered note, an adolescent may evaluate his or her own work performance on a daily basis, with his or her teachers providing summative information based on behavior spanning a 1- or 2-week period.

We suggest that the daily note be faded systematically and slowly. The comprehensiveness of the feedback should be reduced in a graduated fashion. It is recommended that fading begin only after the child exhibits at least 2 weeks of satisfactory behavior. That is, the child should be achieving his or her performance goals consistently across the 2-week time span, and should be judged as exhibiting satisfactory behavior by teachers and parents before the comprehensiveness of the note is reduced. We also recommend that each step in the fading process be instituted only after the child's behavior is maintained at satisfactory levels for approximately 2 weeks. Should the child's behavior deteriorate in the fading process, the consultant should return to the preceding step or to using the original school–home note.

SUMMARY

Although the school–home note is simple in concept, the mechanics of administering an effective school–home note program are numerous and require many skills from the clinician, including consultation abilities, a firm grounding in behavior analysis, and knowledge of classroom routines. This chapter has delineated the activities required of school–home note team members and the consultant across four phases: (1) setting the stage for using the program by selecting appropriate clients and enlisting parent and teacher cooperation; (2) designing a practical and effective program by including target behaviors that are well defined, important, and easily monitored by teachers; (3) specifying reasonable and fair performance goals and providing truly enjoyable consequences for goal achievement; (4) administering the program successfully by providing the student with frequent, positive feedback and continually monitoring program effectiveness.

The chapter has emphasized the use of the six-step problem-solving model as a heuristic for promoting client cooperation and participation, parent–teacher communication, and family contracting. The model is seen as a tool for encouraging all participants to solve problems instead of blaming one another for causing the problem or refusing to compromise. I have emphasized that the model should be used in all phases of development and implementation of the school–home note program. Use of such a model requires the formal participation of all individuals directly and indirectly involved in evaluating the target student or delivering consequences for behavior change.

My colleagues and I view school–home notes as a tool, and care should be taken to avoid using the procedure as a means for initiating punishment, ridicule, or aversive control of children or other program participants. They should only be used with the intention that a feedback system will increase positive, effective communication and socially important behavior change. In this vein, I have recommended that teachers provide children with feedback throughout the day regarding their performance and proximity to goal achievement, and that they should praise children for their efforts and production. It also is important for parents to review the teacher's comments in a calm, constructive, and positive manner each day. When reviewing the completed school–home note, parents should take the opportunity to encourage children's evaluation of their behavior and the actions that produced positive versus negative comments, and to generate solutions to problem situations. Review time should clearly be a teaching time. Consequences should be primarily rewards for goal achievement, although mild sanctions may sometimes be used by parents who can deliver aversive consequences in a calm and predictable manner. The emphasis, however, is on providing children with an unambiguous message: Academic productivity and appropriate classroom behavior are desired and will be acknowledged in truly rewarding ways.

School–home notes are tools that must be used correctly. In order for the school–home note procedure to be effective, the consultant must have a clear, accurate understanding of the factors that maintain unacceptable academic performance or classroom conduct. Table 4.8 describes numerous aspects of developing and implementing the program that are important to establishing effective parent–teacher communication, shaping socially relevant behavior, and establishing powerful reinforcement contingencies. Attention to the recommendations summarized in the table should aid greatly in the development of a useful, effective school–home note program.

APPENDIX 4.1
A Handout for Parents
and Teachers on
School–Home Notes

Home-Based Rewards for Classroom Behavior:
Use of School–Home Notes

DEFINITION

Like regular report cards, school–home notes are a means of evaluating
children's behavior in school. School–home notes are designed cooperatively
by parents, teachers, and sometimes consultants such as psychologists. They
help make communication between parents and teachers more frequent and
positive.

The notes are completed daily by the teacher or teachers and given to the
child to bring home. Parents are responsible for rewarding the child for
satisfactory school performance. In this manner, parents can effectively
monitor their child's behavior at school. School–home notes are used to
increase behaviors such as completing classwork, attending class, not talking
out, and bringing required materials to class.

STEPS IN DESIGNING AND USING A SCHOOL–HOME NOTE
PROGRAM

1. Conduct a parent–teacher conference.

The first step in designing a school–home note is for parents and teachers to
have a conference. At this time teachers should describe the child's problematic behaviors. The teachers and parents should also discuss what they consider to be acceptable and desirable behavior.

In addition to parents and teachers, other people involved in caring for the
child should be included in the meeting if possible. For example, babysitters
and school counselors are sometimes involved.

Both teachers and parents should avoid blaming one another and should
try to make their discussions as pleasant as possible. The general assumption
should be that everyone sincerely wants the child to do better.

2. Define target behaviors.

Using the information discussed, both parents and teachers should define the
classroom behaviors that they would like the child to perform more often.
Whenever possible, target behaviors should be defined in terms of *increasing
good behavior* rather than decreasing unacceptable behavior. This will make

From *School–Home Notes: Promoting Children's Classroom Success* by Mary Lou Kelley. ©
1990 The Guilford Press.

interactions with the child concerning the school–home note more positive. For example, instead of targeting the number of times tardy to class, team members should focus on the number of times the child arrives "on time."

In defining behaviors, emphasize academic rather than conduct problems. For example, "completed work satisfactorily" should be emphasized rather than "worked quietly." Often, when academic performance increases, conduct improves as well.

Do define target behaviors as *specifically* as possible. Clear, objective definitions make it more likely that parents and teachers will get an accurate picture of the child's behavior.

Commonly used target behaviors include:

1. Followed directions.
2. Turned in completed homework.
3. Completed classwork satisfactorily.
4. Used classtime well.

3. Set small goals.

Goals should be small enough that the child is likely to achieve them quickly. This will insure that the parents and teachers have opportunities to reward small changes.

Initially, require only small improvements in behavior. As the child's behavior improves, gradually increase the requirements necessary to receive rewards.

Small goals can be set by breaking the day up into several time periods such as class periods. For example, if the goal is to increase talking with permission, teachers should evaluate the behavior at several different time periods. Or, instead of indicating whether or not the child handed in all homework, teachers should indicate whether homework was received for *each* academic subject.

It usually is necessary to evaluate the child's performance of target behaviors several times during the day.

4. Design the school–home note.

Each note should have a place for the child's name, the date, and each teacher's signature. It is often helpful to leave space on the school–home note for additional comments. The target behaviors should be stated clearly, with a space on the side for the teacher to check whether or not the behavior occurred.

5. Establish responsibilities.

Before starting the school–home note program, the teachers, parents, and child should meet to establish responsibilities. It should be either the parent's or teacher's responsibility to provide the note each day. It should be the child's responsibility to return the completed card to his/her parents. Parents are responsibile for rewarding goal achievement.

6. Set up rewards.

With the help of the child, parents should decide on a set of rewards from which the child can choose one or two when a good school-home note is brought home. It should be very clear to the child exactly what must be done in order to receive rewards. Praise should always accompany the delivery of the rewards. The parents should set up both daily and weekly rewards for good reports.

Daily Rewards	Weekly Rewards
Late Bedtime	Lunch at McDonalds
TV in the evening	Small Toy
Game with Mom or Dad	Trip to the Park
Allowance	

In selecting rewards, it is important to promote cooperation with compromise. Parents should try to reward the child with events and activities that are *truly* important, and should include the child in the selection of rewards.

Although rewarding positive behavior is emphasized, parents may wish to include a mild sanction for poor performance. For example, a parent may wish to require an extra chore to be completed during the time the child would have enjoyed privileges had he or she behaved satisfactorily (e.g., TV, playing outside). Parents should always avoid the use of physical punishment and should emphasize rewards for good behavior.

7. Explain the note.

Do tell children about the program in a positive, constructive manner. They should be informed that the note is intended to help them do better in school and improve their relationship with teachers and parents.

School–home notes are useful in helping a child to understand exactly which behaviors need to be changed or increased. Children's behavior sometimes improves when performance goals are made clear and feedback is provided about goal achievement.

Children usually respond well to the idea of using a school–home note system, especially when parents emphasize rewards for improved behavior. They also are encouraged by the fact that when they do *well*, they will be praised by parents. Parents should point out that without the notes, they would not know *when* to praise or to give privileges.

8. Collect baseline data.

Begin the program by completing the notes for about a week without rewarding improved behavior. This allows parents and teachers to know how the child is performing and is useful to determine small behavior-change goals. During baseline, parents can reward children for simply bringing the completed note home.

9. Provide feedback.

School–home notes work best when teachers and parents provide frequent verbal feedback and praise. Teachers should attempt to inform the child about his or her progress when completing the school–home note. Ideally, feedback and praise should be given on a frequent basis throughout the day. For example, a teacher can inform a child how much of an assignment was completed at the end of the class period.

Each day, the parents and child should review the teacher's evaluations, preferably in order as they appear on the note. Parents should remember to praise children for good evaluations in specific subjects or behaviors.

10. Provide promised consequences.

It is very important for parents to follow through with promised consequences each time the child brings home a school home note that meets the daily goal for a reward.

If the child fails to meet the daily goal or does not bring home the report card, the rewards are not given. Do *not* punish unless a specific punishment procedure has been recommended. The purpose of the school-home note is to set up opportunities for parents to reward and increase desirable school behavior.

11. Fade the note system when behavior improves.

When behavior improves to appropriate levels, the school–home note system should be faded out. A good way to do this is, first, to lengthen the time intervals of each evaluation period. For example, the child may be evaluated two times a day rather than six. Another way of fading the notes is to reduce the number of target behaviors. Later, the child can be evaluated weekly. With a weekly note, teachers rate the child for the entire week and the child can earn the full week's consequences.

If behavior worsens during fading, return to daily notes. If weekly feedback is successful for a few weeks, the child should be able to earn going off the system entirely (but should still receive the rewards). Again, if the behavior worsens, parents and teachers can go back to the weekly notes.

Remember, the key to the school-home note program is *cooperation*. Parents and teachers should maintain communication during all phases of the procedure.

APPENDIX 4.2
Sample School–Home Notes

The sample school–home notes that follow are intended for use with children of varying ages, from preschoolers to adolescents. They also reflect different types of academic or conduct problems. When necessary, notes can be copied front and back to provide enough spaces for class subjects.

SCHOOL-HOME NOTE

Name _____   **Date** _____

SUBJECT_____

    Was prepared for class   Yes No NA   Homework assignment:
    Used class time well   Yes No NA
    Handed in homework   Yes No NA

Homework/Test Grade   F D C B A NA   Teacher's Initials_____

Comments:

SUBJECT_____

    Was prepared for class   Yes No NA   Homework assignment:
    Used class time well   Yes No NA
    Handed in homework   Yes No NA

Homework/Test Grade   F D C B A NA   Teacher's Initials_____

Comments:

SUBJECT_____

    Was prepared for class   Yes No NA   Homework assignment:
    Used class time well   Yes No NA
    Handed in homework   Yes No NA

Homework/Test Grade   F D C B A NA   Teacher's Initials_____

Comments:

SUBJECT_____

    Was prepared for class   Yes No NA   Homework assignment:
    Used class time well   Yes No NA
    Handed in homework   Yes No NA

Homework/Test Grade   F D C B A NA   Teacher's Initials_____

Comments:

From *School–Home Notes: Promoting Children's Classroom Success* by Mary Lou Kelley. © 1990 The Guilford Press.

SCHOOL–HOME REPORT

Name _____   **Date** _____

Period	Classwork	Homework	Behavior	Initials	Comments
1					
2					
3					
4					
5					
6					
7					

Legend: Good = ✓   Fair = X   Poor = O

Parent Comments: _____

_____

_____

_____

_____

_____

From *School–Home Notes: Promoting Children's Classroom Success* by Mary Lou Kelley. © 1990 The Guilford Press.

SCHOOL–HOME NOTE

Name _____   **Date** _____

CLASS_____

    Completed Classwork Satisfactorily   Yes   So-So   No   NA
    Handed in Homework   Yes   So-So   No   NA

    Homework/Test Grades   A B C D F NA

Comments:

_____

CLASS_____

    Completed Classwork Satisfactorily   Yes   So-So   No   NA
    Handed in Homework   Yes   So-So   No   NA

    Homework/Test Grades   A B C D F NA

Comments:

_____

CLASS_____

    Completed Classwork Satisfactorily   Yes   So-So   No   NA
    Handed in Homework   Yes   So-So   No   NA

    Homework/Test Grades   A B C D F NA

Comments:

_____

CLASS_____

    Completed Classwork Satisfactorily   Yes   So-So   No   NA
    Handed in Homework   Yes   So-So   No   NA

    Homework/Test Grades   A B C D F NA

Comments:

_____

Parent Comments

    Consequences Provided Last Night:_____

    Comments About Homework:_____

    Other Comments:_____

_____

From *School–Home Notes: Promoting Children's Classroom Success* by Mary Lou Kelley. © 1990 The Guilford Press.

SCHOOL–HOME NOTE

Name _____   Date _____

CLASS_____

Assignment:

Completed Classwork	Yes	So-So	No	NA
Obeyed Classroom Rules	Yes	So-So	No	NA
Handed in Homework	Yes	So-So	No	NA

Comments: Initials_____

_____

CLASS_____

Assignment:

Completed Classwork	Yes	So-So	No	NA
Obeyed Classroom Rules	Yes	So-So	No	NA
Handed in Homework	Yes	So-So	No	NA

Comments: Initials_____

_____

CLASS_____

Assignment:

Completed Classwork	Yes	So-So	No	NA
Obeyed Classroom Rules	Yes	So-So	No	NA
Handed in Homework	Yes	So-So	No	NA

Comments: Initials_____

_____

CLASS_____

Assignment:

Completed Classwork	Yes	So-So	No	NA
Obeyed Classroom Rules	Yes	So-So	No	NA
Handed in Homework	Yes	So-So	No	NA

Comments: Initials_____

_____

Parent Comments:

_____

From *School–Home Notes: Promoting Children's Classroom Success* by Mary Lou Kelley. ©
1990 The Guilford Press.

SCHOOL–HOME NOTE

Name _____   **Date** _____

CLASS_____

    Percentage of work
    completed correctly   NA   0   25   50   75   90 or Above

    Behaved cooperatively before
    and during class period   YES   SO-SO   NO

Comments:

_____

CLASS_____

    Percentage of work
    completed correctly   NA   0   25   50   75   90 or Above

    Behaved cooperatively before
    and during class period   YES   SO-SO   NO

Comments:

_____

CLASS_____

    Percentage of work
    completed correctly   NA   0   25   50   75   90 or Above

    Behaved cooperatively before
    and during class period   YES   SO-SO   NO

Comments:

_____

Parent comments:
    Consequences Provided Last Night:_____

_____

_____

    Questions/Comments:_____

_____

_____

From *School–Home Notes: Promoting Children's Classroom Success* by Mary Lou Kelley. © 1990 The Guilford Press.

HAPPY NOTE

Name _____   **Date** _____

Time: A.M.

Obeyed Teacher Without Arguing   ☺ 😐 ☹

Completed Classwork   ☺ 😐 ☹

Obeyed Classroom Rules   ☺ 😐 ☹

Got Along Well With Others   ☺ 😐 ☹

Number of Times in Time Out _____

Comments:_____

_____

Time: P.M.

Obeyed Teacher Without Arguing   ☺ 😐 ☹

Completed Classwork   ☺ 😐 ☹

Obeyed Classroom Rules   ☺ 😐 ☹

Got Along Well With Others   ☺ 😐 ☹

Number of Times in Time Out _____

Comments:_____

_____

From *School–Home Notes: Promoting Children's Classroom Success* by Mary Lou Kelley. © 1990 The Guilford Press.

SCHOOL–HOME NOTE

Name _____   **Date** _____

SUBJECT_____

   Completed Classwork

   Obeyed Classroom Rules

Comments:

_____

SUBJECT_____

   Completed Classwork

   Obeyed Classroom Rules

Comments:

_____

SUBJECT_____

   Completed Classwork

   Obeyed Classroom Rules

Comments:

_____

SUBJECT_____

   Completed Classwork

   Obeyed Classroom Rules

Comments:

_____

From *School–Home Notes: Promoting Children's Classroom Success* by Mary Lou Kelley. © 1990 The Guilford Press.

APPENDIX 4.3
School–Home Note Contract
and Record Form

SCHOOL–HOME NOTE CONTRACT

I agree to (daily):_____

_____

_____

I agree to (weekly):_____

_____

_____

If the activities above are performed, I/we agree to provide the following:

Daily rewards:_____

_____

_____

Weekly rewards:_____

_____

_____

Sanction (daily):_____

_____

_____

Sanction (weekly):_____

_____

_____

_____   _____
        SIGNATURE   SIGNATURE

                    _____
                            DATE

From *School–Home Notes: Promoting Children's Classroom Success* by Mary Lou Kelley. ©
1990 The Guilford Press.

SCHOOL–HOME NOTE CONTRACT RECORD

Name _____   Date _____

A good note is:_____

_____

If a good note is earned:_____

_____

If a good note is not earned:_____

_____

If a note is forgotten:_____

_____

If _____ good notes are brought home by the end of the week:_____

_____

If fewer than _____ good notes are brought home:_____

_____

_____

DAILY RECORD OF NOTES   CONSEQUENCES PROVIDED

Monday: _____   _____

Tuesday: _____   _____

Wednesday: _____   _____

Thursday: _____   _____

Friday: _____   _____

Weekly: _____   _____

From *School–Home Notes: Promoting Children's Classroom Success* by Mary Lou Kelley. ©
1990 The Guilford Press. This form was developed by Ginger K. Kendell, Louisiana
State University, 1989, and is used here with her permission.

APPENDIX 4.4
A Handout for Parents
on Star Charts

WHAT IS A STAR CHART?

A star chart is a special way of giving children positive attention. Good behavior earns stars; stars are traded in for other consequences, such as candy, TV time, play time, or a trip to McDonald's. Using star charts allows parents to provide an immediate signal that the child will earn rewards later for good behavior.

HOW TO MAKE A STAR CHART

Here is an example of a star chart parents have used to reinforce a child's good behavior:

STAR CHART FOR KATHY

Days	Make Bed		Take Out Trash		Help Wash Dishes	
	Week 1	Week 2	Week 1	Week 2	Week 1	Week 2
Monday	*		*		*	
Tuesday	*		*		*	
Wednesday	*				*	
Thursday	*		*		*	
Friday			*		*	
Saturday	*		*			
Sunday	*		*		*	

Here, Kathy earned a star for each day she did the good behaviors listed on the top of the chart.

HOW TO USE A STAR CHART

1. Select target behaviors.

When parents are selecting a behavior to include in a star chart, it is best to choose a *positive* behavior. The target behavior can be the absence of a

From *School–Home Notes: Promoting Children's Classroom Success* by Mary Lou Kelley. © 1990 The Guilford Press.

misbehavior (such as tantrums) for an interval of time. Behaviors that occur frequently (such as fighting with siblings or having tantrums) should receive stars at several intervals.

For example, Sally tantrums about six times a day. Her mother has set up a star chart so that the day is divided into three parts—before school, after school, and after supper. Sally can earn a star for *not* having any tantrums during these three intervals.

2. Select consequences.

Parents and children should determine daily and weekly rewards for reaching behavior-change goals. For example, when Kathy completed her chores, she earned 25 cents and 20 minutes of special time with Dad or Mom daily. Larger rewards were provided for six of seven acceptable days.

Parents should attempt to provide truly *rewarding* consequences.

Clearly communicate to the child how many stars are needed to earn rewards.

3. Pair stars with praise.

Whenever star earning behaviors are performed, parents should praise children.

Do praise in a sincere manner. Do allow children to place their stars on the chart if they choose.

4. Give positive attention both right away and later.

When parents use a star chart, a child can get positive attention with a star *right after* a good behavior, and the child can work for special reinforcers *later* by trading in stars.

5. Reinforce every time the pleasing behavior occurs.

In the beginning, parents should reinforce their child each and every time the pleasing behavior occurs. Also, the child should receive a bigger reinforcer when he or she earns stars several days in a row (weekly reinforcers).

6. Reinforce small changes.

Parents should reinforce small amounts of behavior change at first, then gradually increase the amount of behavior change necessary for the bigger reinforcers.

7. Use everyday reinforcers.

Reinforcers need not be extra things, but things parents now give a child noncontingently. Examples include staying up late, watching TV, and playing outside.

8. Keep your promises.

Parents should always tell their child what he or she can earn and with how many stars. They should *only* promise something they can really give the child and should always keep their promises.

5

Special Applications of School–Home Notes

Chapter 4 presents the basic components of a school–home note program as they are commonly described in the literature and used in clinical settings. My colleagues and I have found that elaboration upon these basic elements is sometimes necessary for an optimal outcome. This chapter presents several less common, yet useful, techniques that can be incorporated into a daily report card program. Specifically, the chapter discusses ways of incorporating response cost and overcorrection procedures into the school–home note intervention. Uses of school–home notes with children identified as having attention deficit–hyperactivity disorder are also presented, because these children commonly experience academic and classroom behavior problems. Applications of the procedure with adolescents, and some of the special problems encountered with teenage clients, are described as well. This chapter builds upon material presented earlier. Thus, familiarity with the procedures discussed in previous chapters is essential to incorporating the innovations presented here into an effective, positive school–home note program.

RESPONSE COST

Definition

"Response cost," a technique used for reducing children's behavior problems, involves the removal of reinforcers in response to the occurrence of inappropriate behavior (Weiner, 1962). Operationally defined, response cost is a "punishment procedure in which a positive reinforcer is removed contingent upon the occurrence of a specific behavior, with a resulting decrease in the future probability of the occurrence of that behavior" (Pazulinec, Meyerrose, & Sajwaj, 1983, p. 71).

There are two distinct types of response cost procedures (Weiner, 1962, 1963). The first involves giving and taking away of points contingent on behavior. The second type involves awarding free points at the beginning of an interval and taking away points whenever a targeted misbehavior occurs. It is this second type that my colleagues and I often use in conjunction with a school–home note program.

Although only a few studies have evaluated the effectiveness of response cost in reducing inappropriate classroom behavior, the research suggests that the procedure generally is effective and well liked by parents and teachers (Elliott, Witt, Galvin, & Peterson, 1984; Frentz & Kelley, 1986; Heffer & Kelley, 1987). For example, the procedure has been used to reduce tardiness (Hall, Cristler, Cranston, & Tucker, 1970), inappropriate verbalizations (Salend & Allen, 1985), and classroom disruptiveness (Witt & Elliott, 1982). The procedure also has been effective for reducing inattentive, disruptive behavior during parent-supervised homework sessions (Little & Kelley, 1989).

Uses with a School–Home Note Program

My colleagues and I have used several variations of response cost to promote academic productivity and appropriate classroom behavior. All of these uses have involved awarding free points at the beginning of an interval and taking away points contingent upon the child's display of inappropriate behavior. The technique requires teachers to augment their reprimands by taking away a point or, with younger children, crossing out a happy face. Parents are informed about the number of points remaining at the end of the day in the form of a school–home note. Children, in turn, are rewarded for minimal point loss. Figure 5.1 shows an example of a school–home note that included a response cost component.

As shown in Figure 5.1, the school–home note was completed by Mike's teacher, Ms. Kemp. Mike's day was divided into a number of intervals. Each interval represented the time before and during a specific class period. Ms. Kemp crossed out a happy face whenever Mike behaved in an inattentive or disruptive manner. The evaluation was sent home, and Mike was rewarded for minimal point loss. In Mike's case, he received a variety of rewards when he lost no more than one happy face during each interval in all but one class period. As in any other school–home program, the behaviors that resulted in

SCHOOL–HOME NOTE

Name _____Mike_____   **Date** __3/14_____

Teacher ___Ms. Kemp_____

CLASS_Reading_____

Completed Work:	YES	SO-SO	NO
Used Class Time Well:	☺	☺	☺

Comments:

CLASS_Math_____

Completed Work:	YES	SO-SO	NO
Used Class Time Well:	☺	☺	☺

Comments:

CLASS_Phonics_____

Completed Work:	YES	SO-SO	NO
Used Class Time Well:	☺	☺	☺

Comments:

CLASS_Social Studies/Science_

Completed Work:	YES	SO-SO	NO
Used Class Time Well:	☺	☺	☺

Comments:

CLASS_Spelling_____

Completed Work:	YES	SO-SO	NO
Used Class Time Well:	☺	☺	☺

Comments:

FIGURE 5.1. Example of a school–home note that included a response cost component.

a point loss were specified and clearly understood by Mike, his parents, and his teacher before the intervention was begun.

In addition to the steps for setting up a school–home note program described in Chapter 4, teachers and parents must employ several additional procedures when they include response cost in such a program. A summary of these procedures is presented in Table 5.1. As shown in Table 5.1, teachers, parents, and students should carefully describe the behaviors that will result in a point loss and the rules for losing points. For example, parents and teachers may decide that some behaviors will result in an immediate point loss, whereas others will result in a point loss only after the child is warned (during that interval) that continued misbehavior will result in the fine. Performance criteria associated should be specified in terms of rewards for minimal point loss. In this way, rewards rather than punishers are emphasized as consequences. As in any other behavioral intervention, the performance criteria should be well within the child's ability to achieve. With time, the criteria can be adjusted upward until the child's behavior is similar to that of his or her classmates or is judged to be within an acceptable range.

Teachers should be instructed to take away points in a calm, predictable manner. Children should never be embarrassed or humiliated. When taking away a point or happy face, a teacher should describe exactly what the child did that warranted the point loss. We have found that the procedure probably works best when the teacher softly warns the child that a point or happy face is being removed. When possible, the teacher should walk to the student's desk, mark off a happy face or point, and quietly state why the loss occurred. Alternately, the child may mark out the face when reprimanded and the teacher may initial the recording sheet at the end of the interval. For example, when Mike got out of his seat, talked out of turn, or failed to work consistently on his classwork in spite of a previous reminder, his teacher quietly walked up to his desk, instructed him to cross off a happy face, and described the specific infraction. If she was in the middle of teaching and he talked out of turn, she simply signaled to him to cross off a happy face and explained at her earliest convenience why he lost the happy face.

Another way of using response cost is to provide the child with a number of laminated happy faces that are kept in an envelope by the side of the child's desk. When the child misbehaves by breaking a classroom rule such as getting out of his or her seat, talking without permission, or touching another student, the teacher removes a happy face from the envelope. The teacher approaches the child's desk, quietly and calmly removes a happy face from the envelope, and tells the child precisely why the face was taken away. My colleagues and I

TABLE 5.1. Parent and Teacher Recommendations for Incorporating Response Cost Procedures into a School–Home Note Program

1. *Define target behaviors.*

   Parents and teachers should carefully define the behaviors that will warrant a point loss. In addition, they should determine whether the behavior will result in an immediate point loss or whether one warning will be issued prior to fining the student. The student should be included in the discussions and encouraged to assist in identifying and defining relevant target behaviors.

2. *Determine fair goals.*

   After determining the student's baseline level of performance, parents and teachers should set reasonable goals. The daily work goals should specify how many points or happy faces the student may lose and still be able to enjoy his or her privileges.

3. *Determine rewards for goal achievement.*

   Parents and teachers should establish the daily and weekly rewards for minimal point loss, and specify the contingencies in a contract. Again, the student should be included in the establishment of the goals and rewards for goal achievement.

4. *Make point loss obvious.*

   The school–home note should clearly indicate how many points have been lost, so that the student can evaluate his or her performance in an ongoing manner. Teachers can increase the salience of the student's point losses by requiring the student to cross out the happy face or point when reprimanded.

5. *Accompany point loss with a reprimand.*

   When taking away a point, teachers should provide students with a reprimand, delivered in a calm, neutral manner. The reprimand should describe the specific behaviors performed by the student that result in the fine.

6. *Be consistent.*

   As in any behavioral program, it is very important to provide positive and negative consequences in a consistent manner. This is especially true of response cost. Points should be provided and taken away according to established criteria. Points should never be taken away indiscriminately or out of anger.

7. *Praise frequently.*

   Response cost procedures usually work best when administered within a positive classroom environment. It is very important for teachers to give frequent praise for absences of misbehavior and instances of appropriate work performance. Parents also should find opportunities to praise children for minimal point loss as well as improved behavior.

8. *Encourage children's self-evaluation.*

   Parents and teachers can promote students' self-managed behavior by prompting students to evaluate their own behavior, the circumstances leading to point loss, and ways in which point losses can be avoided in the future. These discussions should be encouraging and generally positive, rather than providing additional reprimands.

usually use this procedure with very young children such as kindergarteners. We have found breaking the day into two intervals (A.M. and P.M.) to be adequate with many small children, although the number of intervals depends on the severity of the child's behavior problems.

We recommend that response cost not be the only form of feedback provided to children and parents. We suggest that the school–home note also list some positive target behaviors. For example, Mike's note also indicated whether he completed his work satisfactorily in each academic subject. By evaluating work productivity, his teacher was prompted to note his accomplishments as well as rule infractions. This information also promoted positive parental feedback when the family reviewed the teacher's comments at the end of the day.

As in any school–home program, it is important for teachers and parents to praise children frequently for exhibiting positive behavior. For example, a teacher can praise a child for minimal point loss and goal achievement. The teacher can and should describe the child's specific behaviors that were incompatible with point loss. For example, at the end of each interval in which Mike reached his goal of no more than one happy face crossed off per class, his teacher described specific examples in which Mike raised his hand before talking and worked diligently on his classwork. Ms. Kemp also attempted to reward exemplary performance, such as the day Mike lost only two happy faces, with a special sticker or classroom privilege (e.g., being the first to leave the classroom when the bell rings).

It is recommended that parents review the school–home note in a positive manner and praise minimal point loss. For example, parents might ask a child about behavior during intervals in which a happy face was not lost. Goal achievement should be enthusiastically and promptly rewarded.

Although parents should emphasize praising good behavior and avoid giving excessive criticism, it often is helpful for parents and children to discuss the specific behaviors that resulted in point losses and alternative ways in which such situations might have been handled. Discussions of point losses should be viewed as an opportunity for children to build their problem-solving and social skills. Children should be encouraged to describe problem situations, response alternatives, and the consequences of each alternative. Parents should ask questions that prompt children to discuss their day and solutions to problem behavior. They should avoid criticizing, threatening, or lecturing, because these behaviors diminish the likelihood that children will communicate in an honest, open manner.

For example, when Mike's parents discussed why he lost a particular happy face, they tried to ask open-ended questions and to prompt Mike in a nonevaluative manner for more information. They also asked Mike in a nonaccusatory manner how he could behave differently in the future and how he might prevent similar problems. When Mike offered solutions, they avoided criticizing his ideas even when the solutions would not be effective. Instead, they prompted Mike to predict the likely consequences if these solutions should be implemented. Since many parents tend to employ a critical style of discussing behavior problems with their children, the consultant may need to give the parents feedback on positive ways to handle this situation.

Children often learn to recognize exactly why they lost a point and begin to anticipate point losses. This recognition and anticipation are desirable and, in our opinion, reflect children's progress toward regulating their own behavior. Often, teachers can encourage self-evaluative responses by asking (as opposed to telling) children why they lost a happy face or point and what alternative behaviors they can perform.

A parent–teacher handout on response cost and sample school–home notes with response cost components are provided in Appendices 5.1 and 5.2, respectively.

Considerations in the Use of Response Cost

A consultant must keep several considerations in mind when deciding whether to include response cost as a component of a school–home note program. The procedure should only be used in classrooms where the teachers manage the students' behavior in a positive way. Ideally, teachers should praise children often for behaving appropriately and should provide reprimands in a calm, unemotional manner. Teachers who are negative and threatening, and who reprimand in an inconsistent, emotional manner, are apt to employ response cost similarly. Attempts to use response cost with such teachers probably will be ineffective and potentially harmful to the program recipients. These teachers usually do best with a school–home note intervention that does not include a response cost component.

Response cost often works well with children who are impulsive, inattentive, or easily distracted. My colleagues and I have found the procedure helpful because teacher reprimands become more salient and effective when associated with important consequences. For example, Ms. Kemp frequently redirected Mike to completing his classwork. When Mike's lack of staying on task resulted in a reprimand accompanied with a point loss, his independent completion of work increased. He stayed on task in order to avoid a reprimand or repeated instruction. In this example, response cost also taught Mike to redirect his own behavior and to catch himself "off task" before his teacher did!

Another consideration to bear in mind is that response cost should not set children up for "bankruptcy." The school day should be broken down into small intervals, and children should be provided with sufficient points at the beginning of each interval, to minimize the likelihood that "point bankruptcy" will occur. The goal should be for children to have at least one point or happy face remaining in the majority of the intervals during baseline. If this is not occurring, then the intervals should be made smaller, or more points/happy faces should be provided per interval.

Prior to beginning a school–home note program that includes a response cost component, it is important for the consultant to review the potential negative side effects with parents, teachers, and the student. The consultant and the school–home note team should discuss the pros and cons of using response cost. The procedure usually increases the potency of teachers' reprimands, is well liked by teachers, and is easy to use. The potential disadvantages and negative side effects include the possibility that the child will be treated more negatively by a teacher, or that the child's classmates will be more aware of the school–home note program when reprimands are accompanied with a point loss. Because of the increased awareness and visibility of the program that sometimes occur, children may be reluctant to use the program for fear of ridicule from their classmates. Many of these potential side effects can be eliminated or greatly reduced by a sensitive, socially skilled teacher who employs the program in a discreet, calm, and positive manner.

OVERCORRECTION

Definition

"Overcorrection" is a behavior management technique that involves the application of aversive consequences contingent on the performance of undesirable behavior. The procedure has been used to diminish or eliminate a variety of disruptive and maladaptive behaviors, as well as to increase appropriate responses (Foxx & Bechtel, 1983). There are two forms of overcorrection: (1) "restitution," which requires the individual to overcorrect the consequences of the misbehavior; and (2) "positive practice," which involves having the client repeatedly practice appropriate actions that are acceptable alternatives to the misbehavior (Foxx & Bechtel, 1982, 1983). Examples of restitutional forms of overcorrection include requiring enuretic or encopretic children to wash themselves and their underwear for a longer time period than is necessary when they soil or wet (e.g., Butler, 1977; Foxx & Azrin, 1973) and having aggressive children write an apology to their victims (Foxx & Azrin, 1972; Sumner, Meuser, Hsu, & Morales, 1974). Positive-practice procedures have included requiring students to repeatedly copy misspelled words (Foxx & Jones, 1978); requiring toddlers to practice a toileting routine 10 times contingent on wetting (Foxx & Azrin, 1973); having aggressive preschoolers practice sharing when they misbehave (Matson, Horne, Ollendick, & Ollendick, 1979); and requiring students who are disruptive in the lunchroom to write self-evaluative essays whenever they misbehave (MacPherson, Candee, & Hohman, 1974).

Foxx and Bechtel (1983) have identified several characteristices of overcorrection consequences:

1. The consequence should require the child to perform responses that are topographically similar to the misbehavior. For example, positive-practice consequences should require the performance of behaviors that are appropriate alternatives to the misbehavior. In this way, use of overcorrection in a capricious, punitive manner is diminished.

2. The consequence should result in the child directly experiencing even more than the effort normally required to correct the outcome of the problem behavior. For example, a child who throws a tantrum and leaves a messy room should be required not only to clean the room up, but to leave it neater than it was before the tantrum.

3. Overcorrection should be implemented immediately following the misbehavior in order to be effective. In this way, the child is unable to enjoy the outcomes of his or her misbehavior.

4. The overcorrection acts should be performed quickly and effortfully, so that the child cannot engage in competing behavior or repeat the misbehavior.

5. The child should be instructed and guided through the overcorrection program. That adult employing the procedure physically guides the child through the response, providing only the amount of guidance necessary to obtain compliance with the overcorrection routine. For example, the mother of a child required to write misspelled words correctly may stand behind the child and guide his or her hand through the response. As the child begins to write the words, the mother provides less guidance. She may first loosen her

grip and then shadow her hand over the child's. Finally, she moves from standing just behind the child to allowing the child to perform the responses with less direct supervision.

Overcorrection has several advantages compared to some other child management techniques (Foxx & Bechtel, 1982, 1983). As discussed by Foxx and Bechtel, the procedure can be very effective at suppressing undesirable responses. Because positive practice requires children to practice appropriate behavior, the procedure may help teach children new skills and thus may serve some educational functions. Finally, overcorrection appears compatible with adults' and teachers' everyday notions about behavior and appropriate consequences, in that the procedure requires the individual to take responsibiltiy for his or her own behavior. (See Foxx & Bechtel, 1982, 1983, for a comprehensive review of overcorrection.)

Uses with a School–Home Note Program

When using overcorrection for remediating academic and classroom behavior problems, my colleagues and I generally recommend that parents use positive practice rather than restitution. For a number of reasons, it is unusual for children to behave in ways that allow them to correct the consequences of their misbehavior. Thus, restitutional actions are often impractical. On the other hand, children can frequently practice appropriate alternatives to their misbehavior; consequently, positive practice fits nicely into classroom and home routines. Another reason we prefer positive practice over restitution is that the former more clearly addresses students' potential skill deficits; children are required to learn and "practice" displaying acceptable behavior. Thus, we believe that postitive practice not only may function to punish inappropriate behavior, but may teach a child appropriate ways to behave as well.

Overcorrection procedures can be incorporated into school–home note programs in a variety of ways. We often use positive practice as a sanction provided by parents when their children behave in a particularly disruptive or inappropriate manner. For example, if a child is caught fighting, lying (including forging a school–home note), talking back to the teacher, or committing some other major rule infraction, we often require the student to write an essay in which he or she describes the following:

1. The inappropriate actions performed and the circumstances surrounding the behavior.
2. The reasons the inappropriate behavior was performed (i.e., the

student's personal rationale) and the consequences of the actions.
3. Several appropriate alternative actions that could have been performed in the situation.
4. The likely short- and long-term consequences of the appropriate actions.

The length of the essay should be developmentally appropriate. We normally choose a length that the child has previously written in school. In general, we suggest that the essay take 30–60 minutes for a child of elementary school age and longer for an older child; the essay should be within the child's ability to complete in an evening. We sometimes require older children who have behaved in a particularly inappropriate manner to write essays over several consecutive days. In such situations, we usually vary the essay questions so that the students continue to put forth effort and thought. Some younger children or children with a developmental delay may be required to copy a list of classroom rules or an already written essay. In this way, a writing assignment is given, but the requirement is more developmentally appropriate.

Having children write essays for major rule infractions has several advantages. First, the punishment is relatively intense but short; thus, it serves as an alternative to the extended periods of grounding that many parents typically require for major offenses. Second, we feel that children often derive a better understanding of their behavior and appropriate alternatives. Third, many parents have reported that they learn about their children and the children's perceptions of their actions through reading the essays. Often, essays bring about increased familial discussion of the situation.

Another form of overcorrection that we use is requiring children who perform poorly on a test or assignment to redo or recopy the work correctly. For example, a child who receives a D or F on a test or an assignment may be required to copy the assignment once, twice, or several times, depending on the type of assignment or test and the child's age. Some of the specific ways in which we have incorporated this type of positive practice into the behavior management program are as follows:

- Requiring children who fail to complete their math assignment to finish the assignment at home as well as to complete several additional math problems.
- Instructing children who receive a low test grade not only to provide the correct answers but to copy the entire test twice.

- Making children write the correct spelling of words misspelled on a practice spelling test five times.
- Requiring children who failed to complete their social studies homework to complete the missed assignment and outline the relevant chapter.

A final way in which we have used a variant of positive practice is to require children to role-play alternatives to inappropriate or ineffective behavior. The procedure involves having a child describe the behaviors that were ineffective or inappropriate in a specific situation, several alternative ways of behaving, and the probable consequences of each alternative. Next, the child and the parent select one or two seemingly effective alternatives based on the consequences and then role-play the selected responses. For example, if a teacher commented that the student disturbed other children, the child and parent may generate several alternatives to the misbehavior and practice the more appropriate responses several times.

Whether this procedure is truly a form of overcorrection or is simply a skills training procedure probably depends on its degree of aversiveness. For example, simply telling the child what response to practice and then requiring him or her to practice the response immediately and often will probably increase the aversiveness of the procedure. In contrast, discussing consequences and role-playing the appropriate responses only a few times will probably not be particularly punishing. A final point to be made is that all forms of positive practice recommended here are applied at the end of the school day. By definition, overcorrection involves the application of *immediate* consequences; thus, some authors might argue that our uses of positive practice presented here are not *true* examples of overcorrection. We believe, however, that the recommended positive practice procedures can be sufficiently aversive that the student will work to avoid them in spite of the latency between response and consequence.

Considerations in the Use of Overcorrection

The most important issues regarding the use of overcorrection are those applicable to punishment in general. As discussed in Chapter 4, sanctions should be provided in a calm and predictable manner. As with other forms of punishment, parents should be told to employ overcorrection only when they have provided their children with advance warning. The consultant should insist that the procedure be used only if the consequences are written into the child's school–home note contract. In addition, the use of overcorrection as well as many other punishment procedures should be avoided when parents are excessively negative or have difficulty delivering consequences in a calm, nonphysical manner. These parents should be encouraged to rely primarily on reward-based programs for behavior management.

Like any punishment, overcorrection can be misused. The procedure should not be cruel or unreasonable for the child to perform. The consequences should be developmentally appropriate and relevant to the misbehavior. For example, the child should not be required to perform the positive-practice routines for considerably longer than it would take to perform the behavior correctly the first time.

Overcorrection should never be the only component of any behavior management program. Research, as well as the dictates of good clinical practice, suggests that the intervention works best when the child is reinforced for displaying appropriate behavior (Foxx & Bechtel, 1983). As such, we recommend that positive practice be a secondary intervention and that the primary behavior management tool be a reward-based school–home note program. We find that a school–home note program emphasizing rewards is not only more ethical, but more effective as well. In our experience, children cooperate better with the overcorrection component of a school–home program when parents and teachers emphasize rewards for goal achievement.

USES OF SCHOOL–HOME NOTES WITH SPECIAL POPULATIONS

Attention Deficit–Hyperactivity Disorder

Description

Approximately 5% of all elementary-school-age children receive a diagnosis of attention deficit–hyperactivity disorder (ADHD). Diagnosis of these children is usually based on parent and teacher reports that the children display significant problems with impulsivity, overactivity, inattentiveness, and a lack of rule-governed behavior (e.g., independent work habits) (Barkley, 1988). Barkley (1988) suggests that the diagnosis of ADHD be based on (1) parent and/or teacher complaints of these behavior problems; (2) scores 2 standard deviations above the mean on standardized measures of ADHD; (3) onset before 6 years of age and duration of at least 12 months; and (4) absence of language or sensory handicaps.

Children diagnosed as having ADHD are a very heterogeneous group. They vary a great deal with regard to the relative presence of various symptoms, as well as the pervasiveness of the symptoms. Children also vary widely with regard to the degree to which they are

oppositional and engage in a variety of aggressive or antisocial behaviors. As one might imagine, prognosis is hardly ever clear-cut.

These children are often treated effectively with behavioral interventions, including contingency management programs at home
and at school; social skills and impulse control training; and pharmacological agents (Gadow, 1988). Some authors argue that a combined
behavioral–pharmacological treatment is often necessary to normal-
ize the behavior of many ADHD children (Rapport, 1981). Because
these children usually display both academic and classroom behavior
problems, school–home notes very often comprise at least a part of
the child's treatment program.

Given the heterogeneity of ADHD children, the diagnosis is relatively unhelpful to the functional analysis and treatment planning. As
discussed in Chapter 3, diagnosing children as having ADHD merely
provides a label that very globally describes a behavioral syndrome.
Instead, some of the more pervasive characteristics often displayed
by ADHD children are setting events that affect subsequent stimulus–response interactions. For ease of discussion, however, some of
our uses of school–home notes with children diagnosed as having
ADHD are presented here in a brief, nonspecific manner. I suggest
that the reader employ the idiographic assessment framework presented in Chapter 3 when using school–home notes with ADHD
children.

School–Home Notes With ADHD Children

My colleagues and I use school–home notes with ADHD children as
both a form of treatment and a means of evaluation. When it is a form
of treatment, the school–home note program is designed and administered much as it is with any other student. The school–home note
team identifies and defines target behaviors that are socially relevent,
occur frequently throughout the day, and are within the child's ability
to change. These behaviors and performance criteria are listed on the
note. After a baseline period, the child is rewarded for improved
behavior. In addition to these basic procedures, however, we find that
response cost is often an important component of the program, given
the degree to which ADHD children behave impulsively. These children often talk out of turn, get out of their seats, or become distracted. For children with these problems, response cost often increases their self-regulation of impulsive and inattentive behavior.
That is, the increased feedback and rewards for behavior inhibition
often result in improved behavior in ADHD children.

One of the advantages of using a school–home note program with

ADHD children is that the procedure can be used to evaluate students' behavior on a daily basis. The data derived from the daily note are useful in determining baseline performance levels and the effectiveness of various interventions. For example, the note can be used to evaluate the separate and combined effects of behavioral and pharmacological interventions. The note can also be used to compare the effectiveness of various contingency management procedures. For example, with some very disruptive children, we employ classroom-based contingency management procedures along with home-based rewards. Finally, data derived from a school–home note are also useful for evaluating the effects of different medications or a single medication (e.g., Ritalin) given in varying dosages. The evaluation of different dosages can be very important, as dosage levels have an idiosyncratic effect on academic performance and behavior. A relatively large dosage, for example, may result in improved conduct but a deterioration in academic performance (Rapport, 1981).

The potential importance of the data derived from the school–home note for evaluating treatment effectiveness should not be underestimated. For many parents, simply knowing the relative effectiveness of various interventions can be of great assistance to them and their physicians in deciding to employ medication as a behavior management technique. For example, a parent may decide to try medication along with a contingency management procedure if the behavioral program alone does not substantially improve behavior. On the other hand, a parent may decide against medication because a behavioral program is sufficiently effective or because daily medication does not increase academic productivity beyond that obtained with a behavioral intervention alone.

The notes also yield some information about the circumstances that affect performance. For example, examination of the data may suggest that a child's behavior deteriorates in the afternoon. The data may also indicate that the child performs better in certain classroom situations than others. These data can be useful in regulating medication as well as in planning behavioral interventions.

Some ADHD children exhibit very serious, pervasive, and chronic behavior problems. For these children, school–home notes can be a very important source of feedback about their daily performance and how their behavior is perceived by others. We have found that this additional feedback can aid in the acquisition of self-control and rule-governed behavior. These children's parents often view school–home notes as the lifeline between home and school. The information is often carefully evaluated by parents and used to plan the evening's homework session. Many parents of ADHD children are faced with the very arduous task of promoting age-appropriate behavior and adequate academic skill acquisition in highly distractible, disruptive youngsters. School–home notes can be used to inform parents about their children's acceptable and unacceptable behavior. The information can be used by parents as stimuli for teaching problem-solving, social, and self-control skills. For example, when parents are informed about a child's rule infractions or lack of preparation for class, the behavior can be discussed and alternative responses can be generated.

ADOLESCENTS

Rationale for Using School–Home Notes with Teenagers

In many respects, employing school–home notes for increasing academic productivity in teenage students seems to go against societal expectations. Many adults believe that teenagers should complete required work independently and that using school–home notes only makes them more dependent on parental supervision. Some adults believe that adolescence is the time to "sink or swim" academically. Some parents believe it is up to teenagers to decide whether or not they want to go to summer school, repeat a grade, or discontinue their education.

Rather than viewing school–home notes as a way of increasing adolescents' dependence on adult-mediated interventions, my colleagues and I view the procedure as a steppingstone to self-management. Through increased parental monitoring and contingent delivery of privileges, the adolescent student begins to function more competently. Our goal is then to systematically fade out the added adult involvement associated with a school–home program; this is replaced by self-managed academic productivity.

For example, we have encountered many junior high school students who lack the necessary study, organizational, and self-control skills for competent academic functioning. Some of these students apparently lack the ability to organize their notebooks, complete and hand in their homework, and bring necessary materials to class. They may bring their English notebook to math class and leave their reading homework in their social studies binder. School–home notes with these students can be an important means of building organizational skills and independent work habits. Although a school–home note program does not teach these students to be better organized, it does motivate them to develop and use better organizational skills. Very often, a student's parents and conscientious peers are more than happy to assist the disorganized teenager.

Recommended Procedures

The manner in which the consultant presents the school–home note program to the adolescent client can greatly affect the student's cooperation with the procedure and program effectiveness. My colleagues and I recommend that the consultant present the notion of a school–home note program to the adolescent privately. During this session, the consultant should encourage the adolescent to discuss his or her academic record, previously attempted methods of promoting academic success, and reasons why the attempts failed. Based on the adolescent's discussion, the consultant can present relevant rationales for using the school–home note procedure. Generally, we discuss the potential advantages of increased academic productivity. One reason why the procedure is frequently advantageous for adolescents is that parents decrease their nagging and questioning about grades and homework, because daily reports provide objective feedback. It is often the case that parents have taken away a good many privileges because of poor grades (e.g., use of the car, telephone, after-school activities). Participation in a school–home note program may be a method of earning back the privileges prior to a new grading period. For example, consider the adolescent whose parents have taken away telephone use and TV viewing on school nights until the teenager brings home improved grades on his or her report card. Report cards may not be due for 6 weeks. The punished teenager often likes the idea of a school–home note program if he or she is able to enjoy watching TV or talking on the telephone for bringing home a satisfactory report.

In working with teenagers, we stress how increased feedback from teachers will benefit them. We point out that it is difficult for many students to develop a clear understanding of teachers' expectations and methods of evaluation. We stress that school–home notes offer a source of objective feedback that can clarify teachers' performance criteria as well as a teenager's own behavior and academic standing. In addition, use of the note can increase teachers' accountability; this can be very important to students who feel they are being mistreated by a specific teacher.

We also recommend that the consultant review with the adolescent his or her personal educational and vocational goals and evaluate the degree to which the adolescent's current academic performance will lead to goal achievement. Based on these discussions, the consultant and the student can collaboratively identify the student's academic strengths and weaknesses and develop plans for improving behavior. This discussion presents school–home notes within a broader context. The note system is only one of the many ways in which the consultant and student will work together to increase the adolescent's competent functioning at school and elsewhere. These discussions should communicate to the student that the consultant is not just one more person making decisions for him or her. Other treatments we frequently provide along with school–home notes include training in study skills, problem-solving, anger control, and social skills.

In mediating discussions of rewards for goal achievement, we suggest that the consultant adopt the role of student advocate. We often discuss with parents ways in which they might compromise or make it worthwhile to the adolescent to cooperate with a school–home note program. For example, we often recommend that parents agree to provide priviliges that have been withdrawn due to poor grades, or reward the student with a desired yet previously unavailable activity. For example, a 12-year-old who has not been allowed to attend a movie with his or her friends may be allowed to do so under certain conditions if the privilege is earned.

After setting up the note program, the consultant should review the teachers' evaluations with the student and discuss ways of improving his or her performance. We find that we, as consultants, are better able to enlist adolescents in discussions of problems than parents are. In addition, we sometimes discuss the completed notes with parents and adolescents together after first discussing the information with the adolescents alone.

A final way to promote adolescents' cooperation with a school–home program is to continue to monitor their involvement as long as the procedure is used. We find that adolescents sometimes disclose problems that they are unwilling to discuss with their parents. We do not necessarily view this as a sign of poor parent–adolescent communication, as most adolescents work hard to maintain some separateness from their parents.

SUMMARY AND CONCLUDING REMARKS

This chapter has presented several innovative ways in which school–home notes can be combined with other techniques to increase children's academic productivity and improve classroom behavior. Specifically, two punishment procedures—response cost and overcorrection of the form of positive practice—have been recommended as useful procedures for inclusion in a daily note program. My colleagues and I recommend that response cost and positive practice, like any other punishment, should be used within a positive context and should never be the only treatment component. The procedures should be used in a calm and predictable manner and should never be recommended to parents and teachers who tend to rely on negative child management techniques.

A school–home note program can be a very useful evaluation and treatment tool with children diagnosed as having ADHD. As a treatment, the procedure is set up and administered much as it is with other children, except that response cost should typically be included. As an evaluation tool, the school–home note provides data on a child's baseline performance, as well as on the effects of any treatment the child may be receiving. For example, the program can be used to compare the separate and additive effects of behavioral and pharmacological interventions.

Although adolescent students may resist participating in a school–home program, we recommend the procedure as a steppingstone to independent functioning. The consultant who sets up a school–home note program with a teenage client should emphasize the benefits of increased teacher feedback. These benefits include the fact that parents' attitudes often become more positive when they are assured that their children are performing satisfactorily; students can use the information to learn about how others perceive them; and teachers are sometimes made more accountable because their evaluations are made more public.

A school–home note program is a tool for effectively managing children's classroom behavior. We believe the procedure offers some advantages over many other classroom interventions because of the emphasis on increased parent involvement. However, daily notes are only effective when used with appropriate clients under appropriate conditions. This book has attempted to describe the clients, procedures, and circumstances under which school–home notes work best.

As in any book of this nature, much has been left unsaid. Although I have discussed some of the problems that may arise when school–home notes are employed, many clinical issues arise that must be addressed sensitively and judiciously. Issues of client resistance, treatment integrity, and response generalization continue to plague researchers and clinicians alike. Consultants using school–home notes are hardly immune to these problems. Thus, I believe that at the core of any successful intervention is an effective clinician who conceptualizes client problems from a broad-based, behavior-analytic perspective. This belief brings us back to the beginning of the book where behavioral assessment was described.

APPENDIX 5.1
A Handout for Parents and Teachers on the General Use of Response Cost

The Price for Bad Behavior:
Using Response Cost

DEFINITION

"Response cost" is a punishment technique. It involves taking away points each time a misbehavior occurs. Children must have a certain number of points left at the end of the day if they are to enjoy their privileges. Thus, misbehavior *costs* children the opportunity to have the activities that they enjoy. Although response cost is a punishment, the program *only* works if children are very frequently praised when they behave in ways their parents enjoy.

HOW TO USE RESPONSE COST

1. Define the target behaviors.

Response cost is a procedure best used for decreasing behavior problems that occur frequently, such as fighting with peers, having tantrums, or getting out of the seat during class. In order to define the behaviors that will result in lost points when they occur, parents and teachers should do the following:

1. List the behaviors they want the child to exhibit less often.
2. Describe exactly what each behavior consists of.
3. Discuss the behaviors with the child so that everyone understands what behaviors are unacceptable.

Here are some examples:

	Talking back:	"Whenever I give Susie an instruction and she complains or argues."
	Fighting:	"Whenever Henry raises his voice, argues and criticizes, or hits somebody else."

2. Determine fair goals.

Before starting the program, parents and teachers should determine how many points the child can lose in a day *and* still be allowed to enjoy his or her

From *School–Home Notes: Promoting Children's Classroom Success* by Mary Lou Kelley. © 1990 The Guilford Press.

privileges. They should set reasonable goals based on how often the child misbehaves *now*. It often is helpful to *count* how often the child exhibits the target behaviors for several days before the point system goes into effect. In this way, everyone can be sure the goals are fair and within the child's ability to achieve. No one should expect perfection!

For example, during baseline, Jeff's mother and teacher realized Jeff disobeyed or argued about six times a day. Therefore, Jeff was allowed to exhibit the behavior three times a day and still enjoy his rewards during treatment.

With younger children or children who misbehave very often, it may be best to break the day into several time periods; each period should allow only a set number of misbehaviors in order for rewards to be earned. For instance, with young children the day can be broken into three parts: morning, afternoon, and evening. In this way, children are rewarded for goal achievement at the end of each time period.

3. Determine rewards.

Both small daily rewards and larger weekly rewards should be given when children lose only a few points and therefore achieve their goals. Daily rewards should be those now available to the child that parents are willing to provide *only when* the child achieves his or her goal. It is a good idea to include several from which the child may choose one or two. Some examples include: TV in the evening, late bedtime, special time with Mom or Dad, and stories at bedtime.

Weekly rewards are those children earn when they achieve their goals on *most* days during the week. Again, it is best to include several from which the child may choose one or two. Some examples include: allowance, lunch at McDonald's, a trip to the park, a movie, and having a friend sleep over.

The child should be included in setting up the reward list. Children enjoy planning activities they will earn with good behavior. Rewards should be changed from time to time to avoid having the child get bored with the choices.

4. Make point loss obvious.

The school–home note should list a series of numbers or happy faces; a teacher will cross out one each time the child loses a point. Also, a line in the series should indicate when the child will no longer earn rewards if the line is crossed. At home, the note should be posted in an obvious place such as on the refrigerator, so that the child can see how well he or she has done that day.

5. Discuss the procedure with the child.

Before beginning to use response cost, both parents and teachers should make sure that the child understands exactly how the procedure works and what is expected of him or her in order to keep tokens or points. The procedure should be rehearsed when the child is *not* misbehaving.

6. Remove points immediately.

A teacher should remove a point immediately after the child misbehaves. However, the teacher may wish to provide *one warning* that if the child does not immediately obey an instruction or stop a misbehavior, a point will be lost. Then the teacher should follow through with the warning within a short period of time (such as 1 minute) if the instruction is still not obeyed. It is up to the teacher whether to give a warning. It is important, however, to be consistent and to give *no more* than one warning.

7. Accompany point loss with a reprimand.

When a point is taken away, the teacher should describe *exactly* what was done wrong and ask the child to repeat the reprimand. Here are some examples:

"George, you lose a point for interrupting me when I was talking. Tell me *why* you lose a point."

"Sally, you lose a point. You did not go to the blackboard when I asked. Now tell me *why* you lost a point."

Describing *why* a point was lost and requiring the child to repeat the reason will help the child learn what behaviors are unacceptable.

8. Praise frequently.

Although response cost is a punishment, it only works when parents and teachers very frequently praise children for behaving in ways they enjoy. An important goal should be to use praise as a method for teaching. When parents and teachers praise frequently, a child will learn *how* to behave. In addition, enthusiastic praise when rewards are earned will make response cost a positive experience for the child.

9. Be consistent.

Teachers should make every reasonable attempt to take away points *consistently* when necessary. They should avoid giving in or giving extra chances.

At the same time, teachers should consistently praise a child for behaving in ways they enjoy, and parents should *always* provide the rewards earned.

10. Another way to use response cost.

Response cost can also be used in a more informal way, which may be preferable for older children. An existing reinforcer or privilege is simply removed when inappropriate behavior occurs. For example, coming home late may result in the withdrawal of the privilege of going out the next night. It is best to specify the response cost in advance when possible.

APPENDIX 5.2
School–Home Notes
That Include a
Response Cost Component

SCHOOL–HOME NOTE

Name _____   **Date** _____

SUBJECT_____

Used Class Time Well   Yes   No   NA   Homework Assignment:
Handed in Homework   Yes   No   NA

Homework/Test Grade   F   D   C   B   A   NA

Number of Times Corrected
Before/During Class Period: 1   2   3   4   5   Teacher's Initials_____

SUBJECT_____

Used Class Time Well   Yes   No   NA   Homework Assignment:
Handed in Homework   Yes   No   NA

Homework/Test Grade   F   D   C   B   A   NA

Number of Times Corrected
Before/During Class Period: 1   2   3   4   5   Teacher's Initials_____

SUBJECT_____

Used Class Time Well   Yes   No   NA   Homework Assignment:
Handed in Homework   Yes   No   NA

Homework/Test Grade   F   D   C   B   A   NA

Number of Times Corrected
Before/During Class Period: 1   2   3   4   5   Teacher's Initials_____

SUBJECT_____

Used Class Time Well   Yes   No   NA   Homework Assignment:
Handed in Homework   Yes   No   NA

Homework/Test Grade   F   D   C   B   A   NA

Number of Times Corrected
Before/During Class Period: 1   2   3   4   5   Teacher's Initials_____

From *School–Home Notes: Promoting Children's Classroom Success* by Mary Lou Kelley. © 1990 The Guilford Press.

SCHOOL–HOME NOTE

Name _____   **Date** _____

SUBJECT_____

  Completed Classwork Satisfactorily: Good   Fair   Poor   NA

  Obeyed Classroom Rules: ☺   ☺   ☺

  Comments:

_____

SUBJECT_____

  Completed Classwork Satisfactorily: Good   Fair   Poor   NA

  Obeyed Classroom Rules: ☺   ☺   ☺

  Comments:

_____

SUBJECT_____

  Completed Classwork Satisfactorily: Good   Fair   Poor   NA

  Obeyed Classroom Rules: ☺   ☺   ☺

  Comments:

_____

SUBJECT_____

  Completed Classwork Satisfactorily: Good   Fair   Poor   NA

  Obeyed Classroom Rules: ☺   ☺   ☺

  Comments:

_____

SUBJECT_____

  Completed Classwork Satisfactorily: Good   Fair   Poor   NA

  Obeyed Classroom Rules: ☺   ☺   ☺

  Comments:

_____

From *School–Home Notes: Promoting Children's Classroom Success* by Mary Lou Kelley. © 1990 The Guilford Press.

6

Case Illustrations

This chapter describes several different applications of school–home notes. The cases are presented briefly, with the primary emphasis on the school–home note intervention rather than on assessment data. We have attempted to include a variety of problems and circumstances. For the purpose of demonstrating the generalizability of the procedure, the chapter includes two case examples (those of Bill and Steve) evaluated, treated, and described by child clinical and school psychology graduate students (Debbie Miller and Ginger K. Kendell, respectively) working under the supervision of a licensed psychologist (Kelley).

MARTIN

Identifying Information

Martin was an 8-year-old male who attended third grade at a parochial school. He was referred for evaluation and treatment because of his inattentiveness, lack of independent work completion, and distractibility. The parents were concerned that he might have attention deficit–hyperactivity disorder (ADHD).

Martin lived with his parents, both of whom were employed and college-educated. Martin was an only child.

Developmental History

According to his parents, Martin's medical and developmental history were unremarkable, with the exception that he had been asthmatic since about 18 months old. The asthma was well controlled at the time of the referral, and he was not taking any medication.

The parents reported that Martin had a history of having a short attention span, being easily distracted, and fidgeting excessively. They stated that they had compensated for these problems by altering their routines in order to provide greater supervision. The parents stated that they enjoyed a good relationship with Martin and that they were able to maintain positive, productive interactions with their son.

Martin's inattentiveness had been noted by his previous teachers. They stated to the parents that Martin required a great deal of supervision in order to keep him on task. However, the mother and father indicated that Martin had never been a behavior problem in school and had always gotten along well with other children.

The parents denied a history of family problems, marital conflict, drug or alcohol abuse, or any other remarkable life events.

Assessment

Interview Data

Interviews with the parents and Martin's current teacher revealed that Martin was considerably less attentive, was more easily distracted, and required greater supervision than the average child his age. They also stated that Martin chewed on his clothes and other objects almost all the time. He seemed to have good self-esteem, however, except that he would become disappointed in himself and sometimes cry when he failed to complete his assignments or tests. The adult informants agreed that Martin had many strengths: He usually followed instructions except when he became distracted; he was well-mannered; he interacted in a cooperative, socially appropriate manner with other children; and he was well liked by adults and peers.

The parents' and teacher's primary concern was to increase Martin's rate of independent work completion in the classroom. They reported that he was receiving above-average grades and that whatever work he completed usually was accurate. However, his slow rate of work production had resulted in his not completing several tests. The teacher also reported that she had placed Martin's desk next to hers because he required frequent redirection.

When Martin was interviewed, he answered questions in a cooperative, insightful manner. He stated that he wanted to improve his independent work completion and to perform well in school. He stated that he liked his teacher and parents, and believed he generally got along well with family and friends. When presented with the possibility of using a school–home note system, he stated that he liked the idea very much and believed that it would help him to complete his work more quickly. He said that he would not mind bringing notes to school or having other children know about the notes.

Questionnaire and Objective Test Data

At the parents' request, Martin was administered the Wechsler Intelligence Scale for Children—Revised (WISC-R; Wechsler, 1974). On this objective measure of cognitive functioning, Martin's Full Scale score placed him at the 83rd percentile compared to other children his age in the standardization sample.

The teacher and parents completed the Achenbach Child Behavior Checklist (CBCL; Achenbach & Edelbrock, 1983, 1986). On this measure, the parents' and teacher's responses resulted in elevated scores on factors indicating inattentiveness and hyperactivity.

Several measures of ADHD were completed by Martin's mother, father, and teacher. Overall, the scores on these questionnaires indicated that the teacher and mother perceived Martin as approximately 1.5 standard deviations above the mean. The father's scores were about 1 standard deviation above the mean.

Classroom Observation

Observations in the classroom by an adult unfamiliar to Martin indicated that he was off task approximately 50% of the time prior to treatment. Several of his peers who were observed for social comparison were off task approximately 8% of the time. The teacher frequently praised Martin's on-task behavior and redirected him when he was off task. She appeared to be a well-organized, effective teacher who primarily relied on positive methods of classroom management.

Formulation

Martin appeared to enjoy good relationships with his parents, teacher, and peers. His primary problems occurred in the classroom, where he was more inattentive and less productive than his peers. He frequently failed to complete assignments and tests. He was not disruptive or aggressive.

The precise contingencies maintaining Martin's behavior were unclear. In part, it appeared that his inattentiveness was a pervasive characteristic that represented a physiologically-based setting event. In addition, it appeared that he had received inadequate shaping and reinforcement for him to acquire acceptable levels of attentiveness and academic work completion.

Rationale for a School–Home Note Program

A school–home note intervention was selected as the primary treatment for several reasons. First, the treatment would provide Martin and his parents with increased feedback about his behavior. This additional feedback would be instructional and could be used to promote Martin's acquisition of self-management skills. Second, the procedure emphasizes rewards for goal achievement; it was assumed that Martin would respond to such a program. Third, the parents wanted more information about Martin's behavior, and the program could provide them with this desired information. Finally, the procedure would provide data regarding Martin's work completion; this information could be used to evaluate any subsequent interventions, including medication if that was deemed necessary.

The Note

In collaboration with the parents, teacher, and Martin, a school–home note was constructed. The note required the teacher to provide Martin with a grade for each class period. The note also included a response cost component; for each class period, five happy faces were depicted in a row. Each time Martin was redirected by the teacher or reprimanded, she was to cross out a happy face.

Response cost procedures were recommended because it was predicted that Martin would respond to increased consequences for inattentiveness. In addition, the parents and teacher were not excessively negative with Martin, and therefore were likely to employ the program in a positive manner.

Procedures

In an initial conference, the consultant described the aforementioned rationales for using the school–home note procedure to the parents and teacher. All team members agreed that the intervention seemed appropriate, and the parents were particularly happy that a behavioral rather than a pharmacological treatment was to be initiated.

The parents and teacher were both familiar with behavioral techniques. Everyone discussed the importance of praising Martin for exhibiting acceptable behavior and implementing the response cost system in a calm manner. The teacher agreed to provide Martin with frequent feedback throughout the day; she believed that it would be convenient for her to do this, given the close proximity of his desk to her own.

The parents, Martin, and the consultant generated rewards for goal achievement and discussed Martin's role in implementing the program. Martin appeared excited about the program and about earning his rewards. His primary incentives were 50 cents per day for daily goal achievement and a special weekend activity for weekly goal achievement. Weekend rewards included lunch at a restaurant or a fishing trip with Dad.

Initially, Martin was rewarded for bringing home the school–home note, although he received additional money for losing no more than three happy faces in four of seven class periods. Over the course of approximately 2 months, Martin's goals were made more stringent, to the point that he could lose no more than one happy face in six of seven class periods and must receive at least a C grade in six of seven subjects.

Results

Over the course of a 2-month period, Martin's performance gradually improved. During the initiation of the procedure, Martin would lose approximately three of five happy faces for each class, although he would do better in some classes than others. Generally, his morning performance appeared better than that exhibited in the afternoon. As noted above, Martin's goals were gradually made more stringent over the course of the 2 months, and he responded by achieving his daily and weekly goals on almost all occasions. Thus, Martin's behavior improved to the point that he lost approximately one happy face per class, although he might have one class period in which more redirection was necessary and thus resulted in his loss of several happy faces. The more stringent criteria were kept in place for several months, as it appeared that Martin needed the additional monitoring and incentives in order to maintain satisfactory levels of independent work completion.

The program was faded and eventually terminated approximately 1 month before the end of school. Martin's initial performance was satisfactory, but deteriorated somewhat during the final weeks of school in the absence of the note, as well as with the added distraction of end-of-the-year activities.

Discussion

This case illustrates the use of a school–home note system with a child exhibiting many of the characteristics associated with ADHD. Although Martin was not disruptive or aggressive, he was very inattentive and required frequent redirection. Given the pervasiveness and chronicity of Martin's inattentive behavior, it appeared that his behavior problems were due to both skill and performance deficits.

His inattentiveness was also viewed as a physiologically-based setting event that influenced subsequent stimulus–response interactions.

Use of the note was associated with increased independent work completion, as reflected by the decreased loss of happy faces over time. According to the parents and teacher, the additional feedback provided by a school–home note system with a response cost component helped Martin acquire self-regulatory skills.

The use of the notes over several months is, in our opinion, a realistic procedure when a child has the type of behavior problems exhibited by Martin. It would be unrealistic to expect immediate, sustained improvements in the behavior of a child whose problems reflect both skill and performance deficits.

The parents and the teacher reported liking the program and appeared to have implemented the procedure with integrity. They stated that they followed through by providing frequent feedback, attempting to use the program positively, and delivering promised consequences.

JIM

Identifying Information

Jim was a 13-year-old male enrolled in seventh grade at a magnet school for students who maintained a C+ average in their final year of elementary school. Jim lived with his parents and older sister.

Jim was referred because of his inconsistent academic performance. According to his parents, he was disorganized, failed to complete his homework consistently, and received fluctuating grades on tests. He was in danger of being discharged from the accelerated program at his school because of his poor grades. The parents stated that Jim's academic performance had become a frequent source of conflict and that their relationship with Jim had subsequently become much more negative.

Developmental History

Jim's infancy, preschool, and elementary years were unremarkable, according to the parents. He appeared to learn things quickly and was an above-average student in elementary school. Although he had always gotten along well with other children and maintained close friendships, he was somewhat shy.

The parents reported that Jim had not been a behavior problem at any point in his childhood. He generally followed instructions and interacted positively with his parents. They stated that most of their conflicts had centered around Jim's academic performance and homework completion.

Although he had maintained above-average grades in elementary school, Jim had a history of being disorganized; he frequently lost papers or failed to bring completed homework to school. Throughout his childhood, Jim's parents provided a great deal of supervision and input to insure that his notebooks were in order and that he completed his homework.

In the latter portion of fifth grade and throughout sixth grade, Jim's grades began to fluctuate considerably. It appeared that his motivation waned and that he lacked the necessary self-management and study skills to function independently. The problems were worsened by the fact that the magnet school program that Jim attended had a demanding curriculum and required much homework. Jim and his parents reported that he had been placed on probation last year because of his grades and barely maintained the C+ average required for continued enrollment at the magnet school. He had been placed on probation again just prior to this evaluation.

Assessment

Interview Data

Jim and his parents reported, as noted above, that Jim was capable of above-average work but that he was very disorganized. He frequently forgot to bring home necessary papers, notebooks, and books. Jim also acknowledged that his notebooks and locker were messy and disorganized and that he had a difficult time maintaining his things in order.

Jim stated that he would like to become more organized and to complete his assignments promptly. He stated that he had become discouraged about his academic skills and had not been putting forth his best effort in recent months. He and his parents stated that they wanted to improve their relationship and to decrease their fighting about Jim's academic performance. Jim's father, in particular, was disheartened about several recent altercations in which he had yelled at Jim and quickly lost his temper.

Jim's academic performance was also discussed with his guidance counselor (who had obtained written and oral feedback from Jim's teachers). It appeared that Jim was inattentive and frequently talked to his classmates during class periods. His teachers described him as needing frequent prodding and supervision to get him to use his time well and to hand in required assignments. As a group, they reported that Jim was not working up to his potential.

Test Data

Jim was administered the WISC-R. Jim's Full Scale score on this measure placed him at the 90th percentile compared to other children his age. Group achievement test scores provided by the school indicated average to above-average functioning in all academic skill areas.

Formulation

It appeared from the interview and test data that Jim's primary problems were lack of homework completion; inattentiveness during class; messy, disorganized work habits; and poor study skills. These behaviors, in turn, produced fluctuating but generally below-average test grades. These behavior problems appeared to be due to both skill and performance deficits. Jim appeared to lack adequate self-management and study skills to perform in a consistently satisfactory manner. In addition, by his own admission as well as that of his parents, Jim did not do as well as he could. He reported feeling apathetic about his schoolwork—a problem he believed was compounded by his parents' nagging and lack of encouragement.

Jim did, however, have many strengths. He appeared to have adequate academic and intellectual skills to perform competently in the magnet school program. He generally was well behaved and got along with his parents and teachers.

Rationale for a School–Home Note Program

The treatment for Jim was multifaceted and included a school–home note program, study skills training, and peer tutoring. A school–home note system was selected as a primary intervention because the procedure would provide Jim and his parents with more information about Jim's daily progress and assignments, which could be used in several ways. The data derived from the notes could be used in a contingency management program where Jim was rewarded for satisfactory work completion. In addition, the data could be used to target specific problems addressed in the study and self-management skills training program. Finally, because the parents would be given information about Jim's academic progress, they would not need to question him about his homework.

The Note

In collaboration with Jim, his parents, and the guidance counselor, the following target behaviors were selected for inclusion in the school–home note: "Prepared for class," "Used class time well," "Participated in class," and "Handed in homework." The behaviors were listed six times, once for each of Jim's classes. Each teacher evaluated whether or not Jim performed the behavior during his or her class. In addition, each teacher was to provide any test or homework grades earned by Jim since the previous school day and to require Jim to write down his homework assignment for the class. The teacher was to initial his or her section of the note upon completion.

Procedures

Each day, Jim brought the note to each of his teachers at the beginning of class. He picked up the completed note from the teacher at the end of class. During baseline, Jim earned daily and weekly rewards for bringing a completed note home. Each day, he earned use of the TV and other privileges. Jim and his parents also planned weekly rewards, which generally involved taking him and a friend on an activity such as a sporting event or camping excursion.

After baseline, Jim earned his rewards for receiving no more than one unsatisfactory mark in five of six subjects. This criterion was made more stringent across time.

In addition to the school–home note and contingency management procedures, Jim was tutored by a same-age peer several times a week. The tutor provided instruction and feedback on Jim's organizational skills and homework completion. For example, Jim repeatedly failed to turn in a social studies notebook that was orderly and contained the necessary papers. Given his problem in this area, the tutor, who was in many of Jim's classes, taught him how to maintain organized notebooks.

Another treatment component consisted of the consultant's reviewing the teachers' feedback daily and generating solutions to minor social and academic problems as they arose. Time management and general study skills (e.g., how to outline a chapter) were taught as well. This assistance was faded with time, so that Jim was required to exhibit more independence in his work habits. Study skills and self-management skills training and general behavioral counseling occurred on an average of once every 2 weeks over a 5-month period.

Results

Over the course of approximately 2 months, Jim's classroom behavior improved to satisfactory levels. At the end of that period, his teachers almost always stated that he was prepared and used his class time well. During about a 4-month period, Jim's academic performance gradually improved and was maintained. Improvements in his academic performance corresponded to the use of the school–home note system as well as the skills training interventions.

The school–home note program was faded after satisfactory levels of behavior change were achieved. Fading consisted of reducing the number of target behaviors evaluated by each teacher daily. The note program was not faded to a weekly system as the school term ended.

Importantly, Jim's grade point average improved by a full letter grade with treatment. His average was 1.7 on a 4-point scale prior to treatment and a 2.7 at the end of treatment. Written reports by Jim's teachers also indicated that his classroom behavior and academic performance had improved during the course of treatment.

Discussion

This case illustrates the use of a multifaceted treatment program with a junior high school student. The treatment consisted of a school–home note system, study skills training, peer tutoring, and contingency management procedures. Although the lack of experimental methodology precludes making definitive statements regarding treatment efficacy, use of the intervention was associated with Jim's improved academic performance.

Several aspects of this case are commonly seen in clinical practice. First, it is very common to encounter adolescents who are performing poorly in school due to a lack of motivation. This case example shows the use of a school–home note system with one such student. Second, it is not unusual to conduct multifaceted treatments with adolescents. We find that many teenagers lack sufficient study and self-management skills to accomplish required classroom tasks. This case illustrates the incorporation of teacher comments into a skills training program.

In addition to his academic improvements, Jim and his parents reported that their relationship was less strained and more positive as a result of the school–home note program. Jim indicated that he felt much better about school and that the program increased his motivation and confidence. Thus, use of a school–home note system provided the parents with information about Jim's academic performance and eliminated the necessity of quizzing Jim about his daily progress.

LAUREN

Identifying Information

Lauren was a 7-year-old female referred because of her clingy, tearful behavior at school and at home. She was failing first grade due to her crying and lack of work completion. In addition, at home, Lauren refused to follow instructions and often behaved in an argumentative, oppositional manner. Lauren lived with her parents and older sister. Both parents were employed full-time.

Developmental History

According to her parents, Lauren reached her developmental milestones within normal limits. Her medical history was unremarkable. The parents reported that Lauren generally had been clingy and whiny both at school and at home throughout her childhood. However, the behavior problems had worsened significantly in the past 2 months: Lauren's classroom behavior had become very problematic after an extended illness in which she stayed at home with her mother.

The parents stated that they were experiencing very significant marital conflicts and that they frequently argued over the most effective methods of handling the children. The mother reported that she was more lenient than the father and that the father was very harsh, although not abusive. The father reported a feeling of being left out of the family, because the children appeared to have a strong preference for being with the mother. The mother admitted that she often gave in to the children and probably reinforced Lauren's maladaptive behavior.

Assessment

Interview Data

Interviews with the parents and the teacher indicated that Lauren spent a great deal of her school day crying, whining, refusing to compete her school work, and withdrawing from her classmates. Lauren frequently asked for her mother and complained of stomachaches and other illnesses. The mother reported that she sometimes allowed Lauren to come home, and, as noted above, might inadvertently have reinforced a great deal of Lauren's behavior. The mother reported having offered Lauren numerous incentives to increase her appropriate classroom behavior, however.

The teacher noted that she also had given in to Lauren a good bit when the problem first began, although she had recently stopped the behavior. She stated that she sometimes attempted to coax Lauren into doing her work and that the attempts were intermittently successful. Both the parents and the teacher felt that Lauren's behavior was getting worse.

Although the parents were most concerned about Lauren's behavior problems at school, because of her lack of work completion, they reported that she had numerous behavior problems at home. At home Lauren frequently disobeyed her parents and cried when she did not get her way. She tended to avoid her father and instead clung excessively to the mother.

At the initial interview with Lauren, she refused to go into the consultant's office without her mother. She began crying and became visibly distressed when instructed by her mother to go with the consultant. Consequently, the mother attended the initial interview. During the interview, Lauren frequently refused to answer questions and behaved in a very oppositional manner.

Classroom Observations

A classroom observation conducted by an adult unfamiliar to Lauren corroborated the parents' and teacher's reports. During the observation, Lauren frequently cried, refused to do her work, and engaged in other oppositional behavior. The teacher was not excessively negative or positive. She did, however, tend to prompt Lauren frequently to complete her work.

Formulation

Lauren's oppositional behavior, crying, excessive attachment to her mother, and lack of work completion appeared to be maintained by multiple factors. With regard to her behavior problems in the home, the parents failed to provide consequences in a consistent, effective manner. It also seemed that the child was a source of much marital conflict and that the parents' lack of spouse consistency and inability to resolve conflicts were major factors in the development and maintenance of Lauren's problems. In addition, the teacher appeared to be reinforcing the behavior in the classroom via her intermittent coaxing and lack of consistent consequences.

Rationale for a School–Home Note Program

Given the multiplicity of problems evident in this family, one treatment approach would have been to begin with more general parent training and/or marital therapy. In fact, the use of a school–home note program in this situation stood a good chance of not working. However, the parents' primary goal was to increase Lauren's work completion so that she would not fail. Given the seriousness of the problems, the parents' and teacher's high level of motivation, and the consultant's judgment that Lauren would respond to a contingency management program, a school–home note program was begun for the child's classroom behavior problems. However, the parents were presented with the formulation above and warned that the intervention might not work, given their degree of marital conflict and parenting deficits.

The Note

The parents, the teacher, and Lauren, in collaboration, decided upon "Completed work" and "Cheerful" as the target behaviors in the school–home note. The behaviors were evaluated during four intervals per day. The performance criteria were represented on the school–home note by a happy, neutral, and sad face for each behavior.

Procedures

The consultant discussed the school–home note concept and the mechanics of using the procedure in separate sessions with the teacher and the family. Due to time limitations, there was no meeting of the whole group; however, all team members clearly understood their roles in the program and appeared highly motivated to conduct the intervention with integrity. During the interview with the teacher, the note was constructed and the program outlined. In addition to completing the note daily, the teacher agreed to provide frequent positive attention to Lauren and to remind her of her rewards on a very frequent basis.

During the meeting with Lauren and her parents, the program was described and the contingencies were defined. It was agreed that Lauren would initially be rewarded for simply bringing the note home. However, it was emphasized that she would receive bonus incentives when she received only two sad faces on any given day. Her rewards included special time with a parent, staying up late, and using her favorite art materials. In addition, Lauren was given a star chart and stickers for monitoring her progress. The parents and the consultant thoroughly discussed how the parents were to deliver consequences in a consistent manner.

Results

The school–home note was immediately successful. Lauren received only happy or neutral faces from the very first day. The teacher reported that during the first few days, Lauren would whimper in the beginning of the day, but that she would quickly begin working when reminded of the rewards she would earn for being cheerful and completing her work.

The parents reported that they administered the procedure in a very positive manner and emphasized providing attention to appropriate behavior. They added that they attempted to provide additional incentives, given the unexpected but extremely satisfying success of the intervention.

Lauren reported that she enjoyed earning her rewards. She freely discussed the rewards she earned and showed the consultant her star chart. She appeared considerably happy and proud of herself for her improved behavior.

The program was faded by reducing the number of intervals in which Lauren was evaluated. At the conclusion, her behavior for the entire school day was evaluated only once per day.

Discussion

This case illustrates a rather novel use of a school–home note program in a situation with many complicating factors. In spite of the severe level of family pathology, the parents implemented the program with integrity, and this resulted in immediate and substantial changes in Lauren's behavior. The parents and the teacher decreased their attention to inappropriate behavior and increased their attention to appropriate behavior. The parents reported feeling much better about themselves and their parenting abilities. They stressed that they appreciated the very direct guidance they received, and that the approach reduced some of their marital conflicts regarding Lauren.

This case also shows that in spite of the multiplicity of factors influencing Lauren's behavior, a very direct behavior management approach was effective. Although a more comprehensive treatment was required to address all of the family's problems, the school–home note intervention did work to solve the specific problem for which it was intended.

After the school–home note program was set up, the parents were taught a variety of child management techniques for reducing Lauren's behavior problems in the home. They were also referred for marital counseling.

BILL

Identifying Information

Bill was a smaller-than-average 9-year-old white male who was in the fourth grade. He was well groomed and presented as an outgoing and friendly boy. He was referred for psychological evaluation because of poor conduct and noncompliance in school. Bill lived with his parents, both college-educated, and a younger brother. His father was employed full-time and his mother was a homemaker.

Developmental History

Bill achieved his developmental milestones within normal limits, and his medical history was unremarkable. Bill had good relationships with both parents and a younger brother. Bill generally interacted well with his peers, but had a tendency to be aggressive toward younger and same-age children. In elementary school, Bill consistently received As and Bs in all academic subjects; however, his conduct grades typically consisted of Ds and Fs. Bill's behavior problems were first noted at the beginning of kindergarten and had continued up until the present.

Assessment

Interview Data

An interview with Bill's fourth-grade teacher, Mrs. Wiley, revealed that although Bill was an excellent student, his conduct in the classroom presented a very serious problem. Mrs. Wiley reported that Bill was never quiet for more than 5 minutes, that he frequently left his seat without permission, and that he often pouted and became very angry when criticized or disciplined. Bill frequently talked back to his teachers and got into fights with other children. Homework and seatwork completion, however, presented no problems for Bill.

Bill's parents reported that Bill often denied behaving poorly at school and frequently stated he did not know why he received poor conduct grades. Bill often said that he was "picked on too much." Further reports from Bill's parents revealed that Mrs. Wiley's methods of classroom discipline were less than optimal. Mrs. Wiley was verbally abusive to the children and inconsistent with contingencies placed on good and bad behavior. Bill's parents reported feelings of frustration because of their inability to control Bill's behavior at school.

The parents reported that, for the most part, any behavior problems exhibited at home by Bill were related to his school problems. Bill would most often display oppositional behavior at home after having been disciplined at school that day. Mealtimes were particularly problematic, because Bill would chew with his mouth open and lean on the table. His parents would have to repeat instructions two or three times before compliance was obtained, and he was sometimes argumentative. His parents reported some marital conflict concerning the issue of discipline in regard to Bill. For example, they sometimes disagreed as to what was appropriate mealtime behavior, and thus disagreed as to when discipline was warranted.

Questionnaire Data

A short screening measure for ADHD was administered to both of Bill's parents and his teacher. A significant score was obtained only from his mother. Responses to an empirically derived measure of childhood psychopathology indicated that Bill was unpopular with his peers and more aggressive than other children his age.

Behavioral Observations

Behavioral observations of Bill during testing and while playing with other children revealed no evidence of excessive motor activity or inattentiveness. Rather, Bill displayed attention-seeking and acting-out behaviors, especially while around other children. For example, he insisted on always being first in line and was very loud in the presence of other children.

Formulation

The information gleaned from clinical interviews, behavioral observations, and test results indicated that Bill's primary problem was noncompliance at school. Although he presented few to no behavior problems at home, other than those that were carried over from school, he exhibited severe conduct problems in the school environment. Although his poor conduct had not yet adversely affected his academic performance, his parents and teacher strongly believed that his behavior problems were likely to produce deteriorating academic performance in the future. His poor conduct disturbed the class and had a negative impact on his popularity. Bill's behaviors in class, such as walking around the classroom, disturbing other children, and talking back to his teacher, seemed to be maintained by positive attention from classmates. Furthermore, Bill's teacher primarily attended to his negative behaviors, which was a frustrating experience for Bill. He received absolutely no attention, positive or negative, when he was well behaved.

Rationale for a School–Home Note Program

It was determined that a school–home note program could serve as one useful component of a comprehensive treatment package for Bill and his parents. Such a program would serve multiple functions. It would provide Bill's parents with more precise and detailed information about Bill's behavior at school, thus allowing them frequent opportunities to reinforce desirable school behavior at home. Second, use of a school–home note would provide Bill with specific information about his behavior. The practice of providing only a weekly conduct grade and no other feedback was obviously ineffective in controlling Bill's behavior. Such information was too vague and allowed Bill to interpret his conduct grades as he wished. In addition, if the school–home note could be implemented successfully, it would decrease the amount of time and energy that Mrs. Wiley would have to expend for Bill. Lengthy telephone calls and numerous meetings after school with Bill's parents about his poor conduct would be reduced by the specific information provided in the notes.

It was believed that a school–home note program would be successful because of the high motivational level of both Bill and his parents. Also, the school–home note would describe Bill's good as well as bad behaviors, thus providing some much-needed positive reinforcement.

The Note

Target behaviors for the school–home note were chosen on the basis of their frequency and salience in the classroom. Those behaviors that were deemed most serious and disruptive by Mrs. Wiley were out-of-seat behavior, talking or making noises in class, hitting other children, and talking back. The behaviors were evaluated by Mrs. Wiley during four intervals per day. The performance criteria were represented on the school–home note by a happy or sad face for each behavior.

Procedures

The school–home note procedure was presented to Bill and his parents simultaneously. They were provided with handouts that detailed each family member's responsibilities and operationalized each target behavior on the school–home note. Bill's parents were instructed to post the information on their refrigerator, in hopes of reducing any confusion or disagreement pertaining to the note. All family members were then asked to repeat their own responsibilities. Mrs. Wiley was provided with the same information and instructions.

For the first week in which the school–home note program was implemented, no contingencies were placed on Bill's school conduct. Rather, he was rewarded for consistently remembering to ask his teacher to complete the notes and for returning them to his parents. Data collected during this first week were then used to determine the criteria for daily and weekly rewards. Daily rewards included activities such as staying up 30 minutes later than usual or playing a video game. Weekly rewards included seeing a movie or having a friend spend the night. These were rewards that were deemed acceptable by both Bill and his parents.

Given the late date in the school year at which the school–home note system was implemented, it was not necessary to fade it out.

Results

Through the final 6 weeks of the school year, Bill's behavior improved gradually. During baseline, Bill earned approximately 60% of all possible happy faces. At the end of the first month of treatment, Bill had, on the average, earned 70% of his happy faces; by the end of the school year, he had increased this figure to 93%. Initially, Bill's behavior was satisfactory in the morning and worsened as the day progressed. This pattern was no longer evident at the conclusion of treatment.

Mrs. Wiley was compliant with the procedure. As the program progressed, it was noted that she positively reinforced Bill's good behavior more often than previously. Fewer telephone calls and special meetings regarding Bill's behavior were necessary, and thus her workload was decreased.

Bill and his parents were particularly pleased with his improved conduct. His parents implemented the procedure with integrity, reinforced good behavior more often, and punished bad behavior less often. They expressed pride in themselves for creating a more positive environment in their home and reported that this change had improved all relationships in the family. His parents further reported that they no longer felt powerless over controlling Bill's behavior at school.

Bill reported that he came to like the procedure as he learned how to behave appropriately. He stated that he enjoyed more satisfactory relationships at school and believed he was treated more fairly. Indeed, Bill reported that he was much happier.

Discussion

This case illustrates the use of a school–home note system designed specifically for remediating a child's behavior problems. This program served the basic goal of improving parent–teacher communication, in terms of both content and efficiency. After implementation of the school–home note program, Bill's parents received specific information on a daily basis about his behavior. They were thus able to monitor his behavior and progress more closely.

Ideally, the school–home note program should have been implemented earlier in the school year. This would have allowed the opportunity to fade out the note, which would have provided a better index of treatment efficacy. As best as can be determined, though, Bill's conduct did improve as a result of this intervention.

STEVE

Identifying Information

Steve was an 11-year-old boy who was diagnosed as having Gilles de la Tourette syndrome. He lived with his parents and older sister. He attended a parochial school and was placed in a generic self-contained classroom because of severe academic and cognitive deficits. Steve was referred by his parents for assessment and treatment of academic and interpersonal classroom problems.

Developmental History

According to his parents, Steve's development of fine motor, language, and cognitive skills was slightly delayed throughout his childhood. His academic problems first became evident in kindergarten. Steve was very disruptive in his first kindergarten class and was placed on Ritalin to decrease his activity level. Ritalin did not alleviate his problems, so his parents transferred him to another school with a less structured kindergarten. Steve attended this school for 3 years and repeated first grade. When Steve was in second grade, he was evaluated for special education because of his academic and cognitive deficits. He was labeled as learning-disabled, and a special class placement was recommended. Steve's parents then transferred him to a private school for children with learning disabilities, which he had attended until the current academic year.

When Steve was 10 years old, his parents noticed a significant increase in the number of tics he displayed (e.g., tapping, twitching, or shaking his hands and feet). After a thorough evaluation by a pediatric neurologist, Steve was diagnosed as having Tourette syndrome and was placed on medication to alleviate the tics. Steve also began taking medication to decrease his activity level.

Steve's academic and classroom behavior problems continued throughout his childhood. These behavior problems included touching other people or their belongings and failing to complete work. However, Steve's school difficulties increased concurrently with his being diagnosed as having Tourette syndrome. These increased behavior problems resulted in his being placed in his current classroom environment, which was more restrictive than his previous placements.

Steve's parents reported that Steve had had four different teachers during his year at the parochial school. All of his teachers had experienced much difficulty managing his behavior. His parents were worried that he would soon be expelled from this school.

Steve's parents denied a history of family or marital problems. No unusual or traumatic life events had ever happened to Steve. After his diagnosis, the parents enlisted the help of a psychologist to teach them to manage his behavior better.

Assessment

Interview Data

Parent and teacher interviews revealed that Steve's primary problems were in the school setting. Steve's parents effectively managed his behavior at home through behavior modification strategies developed in conjunction with the psychologist. They strove consistently to provide rewards for good behavior and remove privileges for bad behavior.

His teacher reported that Steve's behavior was quite variable and that he evidenced four main problems at school: (1) touching other children or objects in the classroom, (2) hitting or being aggressive with other students, (3) refusing to do his work, and (4) not completing work adequately. No specific antecedents or consequences were reported for any of these behaviors. Occasional consequences included lecturing him, making him stay in at recess, making him write lines for punishment, and sending notes home to his parents. Steve's teacher also related that Steve was a friendly and likeable child who generally tried to behave appropriately.

Steve behaved in an amiable and cooperative manner during his interview. He related that he liked school and especially liked his current class. When questioned why he occasionally touched or hit people, he reported that he had no reason for touching them but that he hit them when they made him mad or when he felt frustrated.

Questionnaire and Objective Test Data

To establish where Steve should be placed in his textbooks to optimize learning, curriculum-based assessment was conducted in math, reading, and spelling. Results indicated that he was accurately placed at the third-grade level in reading and spelling, but had not acquired the basic addition and subtraction facts in math. These needed to be learned before he could proceed in his third-grade math book.

To determine Steve's current cognitive functioning he was administered the WISC-R. His score indicated that he was functioning in the mild mentally handicapped range.

Steve's parents and teacher completed the CBCL and the Conners Parent and Teacher Rating Scales (short form) to provide more understanding of his general behavior. Steve scored within the normal range on the teacher-completed scales. His parents, however, rated his activity level at 3 standard deviations above the mean on the Conners. In addition, his parents' responses on the CBCL resulted in elevated scores on factors indicating hyperactivity and aggressiveness. The difference between the parents' and teacher's scores was attributed partially to the fact that Steve was on medication while at school, and partially to the fact that his teacher compared him to other handicapped students while his parents compared him to normal children.

Classroom Observation

Behavioral observation data were collected on several occasions across most of the periods of the day. Steve was on task an average of 65%

across eight observational periods. In comparison, a control student was on task 78% across three observational periods. Three instances each of touching and hitting were observed. One instance of work refusal was observed. Classroom observations revealed a somewhat unstructured, noisy class, with no specific or consistent consequences for misbehavior.

Formulation

Steve's excessive touching and off-task behaviors, as well as his work refusal and insufficient work completion, appeared to be partially physiologically based; they appeared to be maintained by a variety of factors, including ineffective behavior management procedures. His parents demonstrated that proper behavior could be produced through appropriate behavioral strategies. It was felt that Steve might be experiencing problems at school because of the lack of such strategies.

Rationale for a School–Home Note Program

A school–home note program was chosen as the intervention targeting work completion and work refusal. Separate classroom-based interventions—overcorrection and contracting—were implemented for touching and aggressive behaviors. A school–home note system was selected to increase work completion and decrease work refusal because (1) it would involve both the teacher and parents; (2) it would provide the parents with feedback about school behavior; (3) the parents were already effective contingency managers; and (4) such a system would provide an efficient way to alter the target behaviors, as well as to monitor other behaviors such as touching.

The Note

Steve's school–home note was designed with the help of his teacher and parents. The note required his teacher to rate his behavior for five categories across the daily academic subjects. The categories were "Completed task" (which ranged from 0% to 100%), "Refused to work," "Had time left," "Used time productively," and "Touching/ hitting." The latter categories were rated either "yes" or "no." Only the percentage of task completion was targeted to receive a reward. The other categories appeared in order for the teacher and parents to monitor them and receive feedback.

Procedures

The rationale, strategies, and procedures of school–home note interventions were explained to Steve, his parents, and his teacher during separate meetings. Steve's mother was to provide notes for his teacher and provide praise and rewards for Steve. His teacher was to monitor his behavior, provide Steve with feedback, and complete the note. Steve was to remember to bring it home daily. One week's worth of baseline data was then taken. Steve received praise for bringing his notes home during baseline.

After the baseline data were collected, another meeting was held with Steve and his parents to establish the goals and rewards for the note. In addition, a school–home note monitoring chart was developed; this specified the amount of work completion that was needed to receive a "good" note and thus a daily reward, as well as a weekend treat. This chart also provided room to record each day's results. Rewards for good notes were provided daily, and a special treat was planned for the weekend if Steve received at least four good notes.

As mentioned previously, overcorrection and contracting were utilized to decrease inappropriate touching and hitting behavior. The overcorrection included both a restitution and a positive-practice component. The contract specified the maximum amount of touches and hits Steve could have and still receive a reward. These treatments were alternated weekly for 6 weeks to establish which was most effective at reducing his undesirable behavior.

Results

Steve's baseline average rate of work completion was 80%. This was the initial criterion for Steve to receive a good note. After 10 days of meeting this criterion, a new criterion was established at 90% work completion. This criterion was met for 6 of the first 7 days. It was then decided to keep this criterion until the end of the school year. Work completion was averaged weekly, and the average rate of completion for 6 weeks was 92%.

Overcorrection and contracting were equally effective at reducing Steve's touching and hitting behaviors. Baseline data indicated a rate of 4 touches and 1 hit per day. After 6 weeks of intervention, these rates had been reduced to 0.41 a day for both touching and hitting.

The school–home note system was very effective in increasing Steve's work completion and decreasing work refusal. In addition, it was rated very positively by everyone involved. The program was not faded because the end of the school year was near. It was felt that the structure of the school–home note plan would be needed to encourage Steve to complete his work, especially during the end-of-the-year activities.

Discussion

This case demonstrates the effective use of a school–home note program in increasing work completion and decreasing work refusals. It also illustrates how school–home notes can be used in conjunction with other interventions. Steve was diagnosed as having Tourette syndrome and a learning disability. His behavior was quite variable, and his teacher had no consistent consequences for his behavior. His parents, however, were skilled behavior managers. A school–home note program was ideal in this situation because it provided a time-efficient way to increase work completion, allowed all of Steve's problem behaviors to be monitored, provided feedback to everyone about such behavior, and taught the teacher a simple way to change behavior effectively.

Steve's parents and teacher rated the school–home note intervention very favorably. His teacher reported that it was easy to use, and she enjoyed the parental cooperation. His parents consistently established and provided the daily and weekly rewards. They also completed the monitoring form and posted it on the refrigerator where everyone could see it. In addition, Steve reported that he enjoyed receiving rewards at home for his work at school. Thus, in this example the school–home note system was not only effective at increasing work completion, but was viewed positively by everyone involved.

References

Achenbach, T. M. (1984). *Child Behavior Checklist for ages 2–3 (CBCL)*. Burlington: University of Vermont, Department of Psychiatry.

Achenbach, T. M., & Edelbrock, C. (1983). *Manual for the Child Behavior Checklist and Revised Child Behavior Profile*. Burlington: University of Vermont, Department of Psychiatry.

Achenbach, T. M., & Edelbrock, C. (1986). *Manual for the Teacher's Report Form and the Teacher Version of the Child Behavior Profile*. Burlington: University of Vermont, Department of Psychiatry.

Achenbach, T. M., & Edelbrock, C. (1987). *Manual for the Youth Self-Report and Profile*. Burlington: University of Vermont, Department of Psychiatry.

Alessi, G. J. (1988). Direct observation methods for emotional/behavior problems. In E. S. Shapiro & T. R. Kratochwill (Eds.), *Behavioral assessment in schools: Conceptual foundations and practical applications* (pp. 14–75). New York: Guilford Press.

Alexander, R. N., Corbett, T. F., & Smigel, J. (1976). The effects of individual and group consequences on school attendance and curfew violations with pre-delinquent adolescents. *Journal of Applied Behavior Analysis, 9,* 221–226.

Anesko, K. M., & O'Leary, S. G. (1983). The effectiveness of brief parent training for the management of children's homework problems. *Child and Family Behavior Therapy, 4,* 113–126.

Atkeson, B. M., & Forehand, R. (1979). Home-based reinforcement programs designed to modify classroom behavior: A review and methodological evaluation. *Psychological Bulletin, 86,* 1298–1308.

Ayllon, T., Garber, S., & Pisor, K. (1975). The elimination of discipline problems through a combined school–home motivational system. *Behavior Therapy, 6,* 616–626.

Ayllon, T., Layman, D., & Kandel, H. J. (1975). A behavioral–educational alternative to drug control of hyperactive children. *Journal of Applied Behavior Analysis, 8,* 137–146.

Bailey, J. S., Wolf, M. M., & Phillips, E. L. (1970). Home-based reinforcement and the modification of pre-delinquents' classroom behavior. *Journal of Applied Behavior Analysis, 3,* 223–233.

Barkley, R. A. (1981). *Hyperactive children: A handbook for diagnosis and treatment.* New York: Guilford Press.

Barkley, R. A. (1988). Attention deficit disorder with hyperactivity. In E. J. Mash & L. G. Terdal (Eds.), *Behavioral assessment of childhood disorders* (2nd ed., pp. 69–104). New York: Guilford Press.

Barkley, R. A., & Edelbrock, C. S. (1987). Assessing situational variation in children's behavior problems: The Home and School Situations Questionnaires. In R. Prinz (Ed.), *Advances in behavioral assessment of children and families.* Greenwich, CT: JAI Press.

Beck, A. T., Ward, C., Mendelson, N. M., Mock, J., & Erbaugh, J. (1961). An inventory for measuring depression. *Archives of General Psychiatry, 4,* 53–63.

Bergan, J. (1977). *Behavioral consultation.* Columbus, OH: Charles E. Merrill.

Bergan, J., & Tombari, M. (1975). The analysis of verbal interactions occurring during consultation. *Journal of School Psychology, 17,* 307–316.

Bernal, M. E., Klinnert, M. D. & Schultz, L. A. (1980). Outcome evaluation of behavioral parent training and client-centered parent counseling for children with conduct problems. *Journal of Applied Behavior Analysis, 13,* 677–691.

Berowitz, B. P., & Graziano, A. M. (1972). Training parents as behaviour therapists: A review. *Behaviour Research and Therapy, 12,* 308–319.

Bijou, S. W., & Baer, D. M. (1978). *Behavior analysis in child development.* Englewood Cliffs, NJ: Prentice-Hall.

Blechman, E. A., Kotanchik, N. L., & Taylor, C. J. (1981). Families and schools together: Early behavioral intervention with high risk children. *Behavior Therapy, 12,* 308–319.

Blechman, E. A., Taylor, C. J., & Schrader, S. M. (1981). Family problem solving versus home notes as early intervention with high-risk children. *Journal of Consulting and Clinical Psychology, 6,* 919–926.

Broughton, S. F., Barton, E. S., & Owen, P. P. (1981). Home based contingency systems for school problems. *School Psychology Review, 10,* 26–36.

Budd, K. S., Leibowitz, J. M., Riner, L. S., Mindell, C., & Goldfarb, A. L. (1981). Home-based treatment of severe disruptive behaviors: A reinforcement package for preschool and kindergarten children. *Behavior Modification, 5,* 273–298.

Butler, J. F. (1977). Treatment of encopresis by overcorrection. *Psychological Reports, 40,* 639–646.

Carey, M. P., Kelley, M. L., Buss, R. R., & Scott, O. (1986). Relationship of activity to depression in adolescents: Development of the Adolescent Activity Checklist. *Journal of Consulting and Clinical Psychology, 54,* 320–322.

Coleman, R. G. (1973). A procedure for fading from experimenter–school-based to parent–home-based control of classroom behavior. *Journal of School Psychology, 11,* 71–79.

Conners, K. (1973). Rating scales for use in drug studies with children. *Psychopharmacology Bulletin, 24,* 24–84.

Dougherty, E. H., & Dougherty, A. (1977). The daily report card: A simplified and flexible package for classroom behavior management. *Psychology in the Schools, 14,* 191–195.

Dumas, J. E., & Wahler, R. G. (1983). Predictions of treatment outcome in parent training: Mother insularity and socioeconomic disadvantage. *Behavioral Assessment, 5,* 301–313.

Dumas, J. E., & Wahler, R. G. (1985). Indiscriminate mothering as a contexual factor in aggressive–oppositional child behavior: "Damned if you do and damned if you don't." *Journal of Abnormal Child Psychology, 13,* 1–17.

Edelbrock, C. (1988). Informant reports. In E. S. Shapiro & T. R. Kratochwill (Eds.), *Behavioral assessment in schools: Conceptual foundations and practical applications* (pp. 351–383). New York: Guilford Press.

Edelbrock, C., & Achenbach, T. M. (1984). The Teacher Version of the Child Behavior Profile: I. Boys aged 6–11. *Journal of Consulting and Clinical Psychology, 52,* 207–217.

Elliott, S. N. (1988). Children's acceptability of classroom interventions for misbehavior: Findings and methodological considerations. *Journal of School Psychology, 24,* 23–25.

Elliott, S. N., & Piersel, W. C. (1982). Direct assessment of reading skills: An approach which links assessment to intervention. *School Psychology Review, 11,* 257–280.

Elliott, S. N., Witt, J. C., Galvin, G., & Peterson, R. (1984). Acceptability of positive and reductive behavioral interventions: Factors that influence teachers' decisions. *Journal of School Psychology, 22,* 353–360.

Eyberg, S. M., & Robinson, E. A. (1983). Conduct problem behavior: Standardization of a behavioral rating scale with adolescents. *Journal of Clinical Child Psychology, 12,* 347–354.

Eyberg, S. M., & Ross, A. W. (1978). Assessment of child behavior problems: The validation of a new inventory. *Journal of Clinical Child Psychology, 7,* 113–116.

Feld, J. K., Bergan, J. R., & Stone, C. A. (1987). Behavioral consultation. In C. A. Maher & S. G. Forman (Eds.), *A behavioral approach to education of children and youth* (pp. 183–219). Hillsdale, NJ: Erlbaum.

Ferritor, D. E., Buckholdt, D., Hamblin, R. L., & Smith, L. (1972). The noneffects of contingent reinforcement for attending behavior on work accomplished. *Journal of Applied Behavior Analysis, 5,* 7–17.

Forehand, R. (1987). Parental roles in childhood psychopathology. In C. L. Frame & J. L. Matson (Eds.), *Handbook of assessment in childhood psychopathology* (pp. 489–507). New York: Plenum Press.

Forehand, R., Brody, G., & Smith, K. (1986). Contributions of child behaviour and marital dissatisfaction to maternal perceptions of child maladjustment. *Behaviour Research and Therapy, 24,* 44–48.

Forehand, R., & King, H. E. (1977). Noncompliant children. *Behavior Modification, 1,* 93–108.

Forehand, R. L., & McMahon, R. J. (1981). *Helping the noncompliant child: A clinician's guide to parent training.* New York: Guilford Press.

Foxx, R. M., & Azrin, N. H. (1972). Restitution: A method of eliminating aggressive-disruptive behaviour of retarded and brain damaged patients. *Behaviour Research and Therapy, 10,* 15–27.

Foxx, R. M., & Azrin, N. H. (1973). The elimination of autistic self-stimulatory behavior by overcorrection. *Journal of Applied Behavior Analysis, 6,* 1–14.

Foxx, R. M., & Bechtel, D. R. (1982). Overcorrection. In M. Hersen, R. Eisler, & P. Miller (Eds.), *Progress in behavior modification* (Vol. 13, pp. 227–288). Newbury Park, CA: Sage.

Foxx, R. M., & Bechtel, D. R. (1983). Overcorrection: A review and analysis. In S. Axelrod & J. Apsche (Eds.), *The effects of punishment on human behavior* (pp. 144–220). New York: Academic Press.

Foxx, R. M., & Jones, J. R. (1978). A remediation program for increasing the spelling achievement of elementary and junior high school students. *Behavior Modification, 2,* 211–230.

Frentz, C., & Kelley, M. L. (1986). Parents' acceptance of reductive treatment methods: The influence of problem severity and perception of child behavior. *Behavior Therapy, 17,* 75–81.

Fuchs, C. S., & Fuchs, D. (1986). Curriculum-based assessment of progress toward long-term and short-term goals. *Journal of Special Education, 20,* 69–82.

Funderburk, B. W., & Eyberg, S. M. (1989). *Standardization of a school behavior rating scale with preschool children.* Unpublished manuscript, University of Florida.

Furey, W., & Forehand, R. (1984). Maternal satisfaction with clinic-referred children: Assessment by use of a single subject methodology. *Journal of Behavioral Assessment, 5,* 345–355.

Gadow, K. D. (1988). Attention deficit disorder and hyperactivity. In J. L. Matson (Ed.), *Handbook of treatment approaches in child psychopathology* (pp. 215–247). New York: Plenum Press.

Goyette, C. H., Conners, C. K., & Ulrich, R. F. (1978). Normative data on revised Conners Parent and Teacher Rating Scales. *Journal of Abnormal Child Psychology, 6,* 221–236.

Gresham, F. M. (1984). Behavioral interviews in school psychology: Issues in psychometric adequacy and research. *School Psychology Review, 14,* 495–509.

Gresham, F. M., & Davis, C. J. (1988). Behavioral interviews with teachers and parents. In E. S. Shapiro & T. R. Kratochwill (Eds.), *Behavioral assessment in schools: Conceptual foundations and practical applications* (pp. 455–493). New York: Guilford Press.

Gresham, F. M., & Elliott, S. N. (in press). *Social Skills Rating System.* Circle Pines, MN: American Guidance Service.

Gresham, F. M., Elliott, S. N., & Evans, S. (in press). *Multidimensional Self-Concept Scale.* Circle Pines, MN: American Guidance Service.

Gresham, F. M., & Lemanek, K. L. (1987). Parent education. In C. A. Maher & S. G. Forman (Eds.), *Providing effective educational services in school organizations: A behavioral approach.* (pp. 153–181). Hillsdale, NJ: Erlbaum.

Guidubaldi, J. (1982). Transcending future shock: Invariant principles for school psychology. *School Psychology Review, 11,* 127–131.

Gutkin, T. B., Clark, J. H., & Achenbaum, M. (1985). Impact of organizational variables in the delivery of school-based consultation services: A comparative case study approach. *School Psychology Review, 14,* 230–235.

Gutkin, T. B., & Curtis, M. J. (1982). School-based consultation: Theory and techniques. In C. R. Reynolds & T. B. Gutkin (Eds.), *The handbook of school psychology* (pp. 796–828). New York: Wiley.

Hall, R. V., Cristler, C., Cranston, S., & Tucker, B. (1970). Teachers and parents as researchers using multiple baseline techniques. *Journal of Applied Behavior Analysis, 3,* 247–255.

Hartmann, D. P., Roper, B. L., & Bradford, D. C. (1979). Source relationships between behavioral and traditional assessment. *Journal of Behavioral Assessment, 1,* 3–21.

Hawryluk, M. K., & Smallwood, D. L. (1986). Assessing and addressing consultee variables in school-based behavioral consultation. *School Psychology Review, 15,* 519–528.

Heaton, R. C., Safer, D. J., Allen, R. P., Spinnato, N. C., & Prumo, F. M. (1976). A motivational environment for behaviorally deviant junior high school students. *Journal of Abnormal Child Psychology, 4,* 263–275.

Heffer, R., & Kelley, M. L. (1987). Mother's acceptance of behavioral interventions for children: The influence of parent race and income. *Behavior Therapy, 2,* 153–163.

Hoge, R. D., & Andrews, D. A. (1987). Enhancing academic performance: Issues in target selection. *School Psychology Review, 16,* 228–238.

Imber, S. C., Imber, R. B., & Rothstein, C. (1979). Modifying independent work habits: An effective teacher-parent communication program. *Exceptional Children, 45,* 218–221.

Karraker, R. J. (1972). Increasing academic performance through home-managed contingency programs. *Journal of School Psychology, 2,* 173–179.

Kelley, M. L., & Carper, L. B. (1988). The Mothers' Activity Checklist: An instrument for assessing pleasant and unpleasant events. *Behavioral Assessment, 10,* 331–341.

Kelley, M. L., & Drabman, R. S. (in press). Psychological contributions to primary pediatric health care. In D. G. Byrne & G. R. Caddy (Eds.), *Behavioral medicine: International perspectives* (Vol. 2). Norwood, NJ: Ablex.

Kelley, M. L., Embry, L. H., & Baer, D. M. (1979). Skills for child management and family support: Training parents for maintenance. *Behavior Modification, 3,* 373–396.

Kirby, F. D., & Shields, F. (1972). Modification of arithmetic response rate and attending behavior in a seventh grade student. *Journal of Applied Behavior Analysis, 5*, 29–84.

Kovacs, M. (1981). *The Children's Depression Inventory: A self-rated depression scale for school-age youngsters.* Unpublished manuscript, University of Pittsburgh.

Kovacs, M., & Beck, A. T. (1977). An empirical–clinical approach toward a definition of childhood depression. In J. G. Shulterbrandt & A. Raskin (Eds.), *Depression in childhood: Diagnosis, treatment, and conceptual models* (pp. 1–25). New York: Raven Press.

Lachar, D. (1982). *Personality Inventory for Children (PIC): Revised format manual supplement.* Los Angeles: Western Psychological Services.

Lahey, B. B., Gendrich, J. G., Gendrich, S. I., Schnelle, J. F., Gant, D. S., & McNees, M. P. (1977). An evaluation of daily report cards with minimal teacher and parent contacts as an efficient method of classroom intervention. *Behavior Modification, 1*, 381–394.

Little, L. M., & Kelley, M. L. (1989). The efficacy of response cost procedures for reducing children's noncompliance to parental instructions. *Behavior Therapy, 20*, 525–534.

Long, J. D., & Williams, R. L. (1973). The comparative effectiveness of group and individually contingent free time with inner-city junior high school students. *Journal of Applied Behavior Analysis, 6*, 465–474.

MacDonald, W. S., Gallimore, R., & MacDonald, G. (1970). Contingency counseling by school personnel: An economical model of intervention. *Journal of Applied Behavior Analysis, 3*, 175–182.

MacPherson, E. M., Candee, B. L., & Hohman, R. J. (1974). A comparison of three methods for eliminating disruptive lunchroom behavior. *Journal of Applied Behavior Analysis, 7*, 287–297.

Mash, E. J., Hamerlynck, L. A., & Handy, L. C. (Eds.). (1976). *Behavior modification and families.* New York: Brunner/Mazel.

Mash, E. J., & Terdal, L. G. (1988). Behavioral assessment of child and family disturbance. In E. J. Mash & L. G. Terdal (Eds.), *Behavioral assessment of childhood disorders* (2nd ed., pp. 3–68). New York: Guilford Press.

Matson, J. L., Horne, A. M., Ollendick, D. G., & Ollendick, T. H. (1979). Overcorrection: A further evaluation of restitution and positive practice. *Journal of Behavior Therapy and Experimental Psychiatry, 10*, 295–298.

McAllister, L. W., Stachowiak, J. G., Baer, D. M., & Conderman, L. (1969). The application of operant conditioning techniques in a secondary school classroom. *Journal of Applied Behavior Analysis, 2*, 277–285.

Moos, R. H., & Moos, B. S. (1976). A typology of family social environments. *Family Process, 15*, 357–371.

Moos, R. H., & Moos, B. S. (1983). Clinical applications of the Family Environment Scale. In E. E. Filsinger (Ed.), *Marriage and family assessment: A sourcebook for family therapy* (pp. 253–273). Beverly Hills, CA: Sage.

Moreland, F. R., Schwebel, A. T., Beck, S., & Wells, R. (1982). Parents as therapists: A review of the behavior therapy parent training literature— 1975–1981. *Behavior Modification, 6*, 250–276.

O'Dell, S. L. (1974). Training parents in behavior modification: A review. *Psychological Bulletin, 81,* 418–433.

O'Leary, K. D., Romanczyk, R. G., Kass, R. E., Dietz, A., & Santogrossi, D. (1979). *Procedures for classroom observation of teachers and children.* Stony Brook: State University of New York at Stony Brook, Department of Psychology.

Patterson, G. R., Chamberlain, P., & Reid, J. B. (1982). A comparative evaluation of a parent-training program. *Behavior Therapy, 13,* 638–650.

Pazulinec, R., Meyerrose, M., & Sajwaj, T. (1983). Punishment via response cost. In S. Axelrod & J. Apsche (Eds.), *The effects of punishment on human behavior* (pp. 71–86). New York: Academic Press.

Pelham, W. E. (1984). *Behavior therapy, behavioral assessment, and psychostimulant medication in the treatment of attention deficit disorders: An interactive approach.* Paper presented at the Fourth Annual High Point Hospital Conference on Attention Deficit Disorders: New Directions in Attention Deficit and Conduct Disorders, Toronto.

Pelham, W. E., Atkins, M. S., Murphy, H. A., & White, K. S. (1981, November). Operationalization and validation of attention deficit disorders. In W. Pelham (Chair), *Toward objective diagnosis of hyperactivity and attention deficit disorders.* Symposium conducted at the annual meeting of the Association for Advancement of Behavior Therapy, Toronto.

Pelham, W. E., Schndler, R. W., Bologna, N. C., & Contreras, J. A. (1980). Behavioral and stimulant treatment of hyperactive children: A therapy study with methylphenidate probes on a within-subject design. *Journal of Applied Behavior Analysis, 13,* 221–236.

Piers, E. V., & Harris, D. B. (1964). *A manual for the Piers–Harris Self-Concept Scale.* Nashville, TN: Counselor Recordings and Tests.

Porterfield, J. K., Herbert-Jackson, E., & Risley, T. R. (1976). Contingent observation: An effective and acceptable procedure for reducing disruptive behavior of young children in group settings. *Journal of Applied Behavior Analysis, 9,* 55–64.

Prinz, R. J., Foster, S. L., Kent, R. N., & O'Leary, K. D. (1979). Multivariate assessment of conflict in distressed and nondistressed mother–adolescent dyads. *Journal of Applied Behavior Analysis, 12,* 691–700.

Quay, H. C., & Peterson, D. R. (1967). *Manual for the Behavior Problem Checklist.* Urbana: University of Illinois.

Rapport, M. D. (1981). Attention deficit disorder with hyperactivity. In M. Hersen & V. B. Van Hassett (Eds.), *Behavior therapy with children and adolescents: A clinical approach* (pp. 325–361). New York: Wiley.

Redd, W. H., & Rusch, F. R. (1985). Behavioral analysis in behavioral medicine. *Behavior Modification, 9,* 131–154.

Reisinger, J. J., Ora, J. D., & Frangia, G. W. (1976). Parents as change agents for their children: A review. *Journal of Community Psychology, 4,* 103–123.

Reynolds, C. R., & Richmond, B. O. (1978). "What I think and feel": A revised measure of children's manifest anxiety. *Journal of Abnormal Child Psychology, 6,* 271–280.

Reynolds, W. M., & Coats, K. I. (1985). A comparison of cognitive-behavioral therapy and relaxation training for the treatment of depression in adolescents. *Journal of Consulting and Clinical Psychology, 54,* 653–685.

Robin, A. L., & Foster, S. L. (1984). Problem-solving communication training: A behavioral–family systems approach to parent–adolescent conflict. In P. Karoly & J. J. Steffen (Eds.), *Adolescent behavior disorders: Foundations and contemporary concerns* (pp. 195–240). Lexington, MA: D. C. Heath.

Robin, A. L., & Foster, S. L. (1989). *Negotiating parent–adolescent conflict: A behavioral family systems approach* (pp. 193–194). New York: Guilford Press.

Robinson, E. A., Eyberg, S. M., & Ross, A. W. (1980). Inventory of child problem behaviors: The standardization of an inventory of child conduct problem behaviors. *Journal of Clinical Child Psychology, 9,* 22–28.

Salend, S. J., & Allen, E. M. (1985). Comparative effects of externally managed and self-managed response cost systems on inappropriate classroom behavior. *Journal of School Psychology, 23,* 59–67.

Saudargas, R. A. (1982). *Student–Teacher Observation Code.* Knoxville: University of Tennessee Press.

Saudargas, R. A., Madsen, C. H., & Scott, J. W. (1977). Differential effects of fixed- and variable-time feedback on production rates of elementary school children. *Journal of Applied Behavior Analysis, 10,* 673–678.

Schaughency, E. A., Walker, J., & Lahey, B. B. (1988). Attention deficit disorder and hyperactivity: Psychological therapies. In J. Matson (Ed.), *Handbook of treatment approaches in childhood psychopathology* (pp. 195–213). New York: Plenum Press.

Schumaker, J. B., Hovell, M. F., & Sherman, J. A. (1977). An analysis of daily report cards and parent-managed privileges in the improvement of adolescents' classroom performance. *Journal of Applied Behavior Analysis, 10,* 449–464.

Shapiro, E. S. (1988). Behavioral assessment. In J. C. Witt, S. N. Elliott, & F. M. Gresham (Eds.), *Handbook of behavior therapy in education* (pp. 67–98). New York: Plenum Press.

Shapiro, E. S., & Kratochwill, T. R. (Eds.). (1988). *Behavioral assessment in schools: Conceptual foundations and practical applications.* New York: Guilford Press.

Shapiro, E. S., & Lentz, F. E., Jr. (1986). Behavioral assessment of academic skills. In T. R. Kratochwill (Ed.), *Advances in school psychology* (Vol. 5, pp. 87–139). Hillsdale, NJ: Erlbaum.

Shoiock, G. (1978). *Normative data on homework problems of elementary school children.* Unpublished manuscript, State University of New York at Stony Brook.

Spanier, G. B. (1976). Measuring dyadic adjustment: New scales for assessing the quality of marriage and similar dyads. *Journal of Marriage and the Family, 38,* 15–27.

Stumphauzer, J. S. (1976). Elimination of stealing by self-reinforcement of alternative behavior and family contracting. *Journal of Behavior Therapy and Experimental Psychiatry, 7,* 265–268.

Sumner, J. H., Meuser, S. T., Hsu, T., & Morales, R. G. (1974). Overcorrection treatment for radical reduction of aggressive disruptive behavior in institutionalized mental patients. *Psychological Reports, 35,* 655–662.

Todd, D. D., Scott, R. B., Bostow, E., & Alexander, S. B. (1976). Modification of excessive inappropriate classroom behavior of two elementary school students using home-based consequences and daily report card procedures. *Journal of Applied Behavior Analysis, 9,* 106.

Turco, T. L., & Elliott, S. N. (1986). Students' acceptability ratings of interventions for classroom misbehaviors: A developmental study of well-behaving and misbehaving youth. *Journal of Psychoeducational Assessment, 4,* 281–289.

Wagner, R. F., & Guyer, B. D. (1971). Maintenance of discipline through increasing children's span of attending by means of a token economy. *Psychology in the Schools, 8,* 285–289.

Wahler, R. G. (1980). The insular mother: Her problems in parent–child treatment. *Journal of Applied Behavior Analysis, 13,* 273–294.

Wahler, R. G., & Afton, A. D. (1980). Attentional processes in insular and non-insular mothers: Some differences in their summary reports about child problem behavior. *Child Behavior Therapy, 2,* 25–41.

Wahler, R. G., & Fox, J. J. (1980). Solitary toy play and time out: A family treatment package for children with aggressive and oppositional behavior. *Journal of Applied Behavior Analysis, 13,* 23–39.

Wahler, R. G., House, A. E., & Stambaugh, E. E. (1976). *Ecological assessment for child problem behavior: A clinical package for home, school, and institutional settings.* New York: Pergamon Press.

Wechsler, D. (1974). *Manual for the Wechsler Intelligence Scale for Children— Revised.* New York: Psychological Corporation.

Weiner, H. (1962). Some effects of response cost upon human operant behavior. *Journal of the Experimental Analysis of Behavior, 5,* 201–208.

Weiner, H. (1963). Response cost and the aversive control of human operant behavior. *Journal of the Experimental Analysis of Behavior, 6,* 415–421.

Werry, J. S., & Sprague, R. S. (1968). Hyperactivity. In C. G. Costello (Ed.), *Symptoms of psychopathology* (pp. 397–417). New York: Wiley.

Winett, R. A., & Winkler, R. C. (1972). Current behavior modification in the classroom: Be still, be quiet, be docile. *Journal of Applied Behavior Analysis, 5,* 499–504.

Wirt, R. D., Lachar, D., Klinedinst, J. K., & Seat, P. D. (1977). *Multidimensional description of child personality: A manual for the Personality Inventory for Children.* Los Angeles: Western Psychological Services.

Witt, J. C., & Bartlett, B. J. (1982). School psychologists as knowledge-linkers in the solution of children's reading problems. *School Psychology Review, 11,* 221–228.

Witt, J. C., Cavell, T. A., Heffer, R. W., Carey, M. P., & Martens, B. K. (1988). Child self-report: Interviewing techniques and rating scales. In E. S. Shapiro & T. R. Kratochwill (Eds.), *Behavioral assessment in schools: Conceptual foundations and practical applications* (pp. 384–454). New York: Guilford Press.

Witt, J. C., & Elliott, S. N. (1982). The response cost lottery: A time efficient and effective classroom intervention. *Journal of School Psychology, 20,* 155–161.

Witt, J. C., & Elliott, S. N. (1983). Assessment in behavioral consultation: The initial interview. *School Psychology Review, 12,* 42–49.

Witt, J. C., Elliott, S. N., Gresham, F. M., & Kramer, J. J. (1988). *Assessment of special children.* Glenview, IL: Scott, Foresman.

Witt, J. C., Martens, B. K., & Elliott, S. N. (1984). Factors affecting teachers' judgements of the acceptability of behavioral interventions: Time involvement, behavior problem severity, and type of intervention. *Behavior Therapy, 15,* 204–209.

Wolf, M. M. (1978). Social validity: The case for subjective measurement, or how applied behavior analysis is finding its heart. *Journal of Applied Behavior Analysis, 11,* 203–214.

Index

Academic behaviors, 11, 12, 14–20
  in adolescents, 148
  in case illustration, 163–168
  in children with attention-deficit–
    hyperactivity disorder, 148
  direct assessment of, 34, 35, 59
  and response cost, 134
  and skills deficits, 34
  as target behavior, 15, 16, 78, 79
Achenbach, T. M., 51–55, 160
Achenbaum, M., 35
Achievement tests, 58
Acting out behavior, 173
Adolescent Activity Checklist, 52
Adolescents, 14, 17, 148–150
  and changes in contingency contract,
    104
  and communications guidelines, 86, 87
  depression in, 45
  and school–home notes program, 68,
    81, 96, 148–150, 151, 165–168
  self-monitoring in, 111, 148
  self-report instruments for, 51, 52, 55
Afton, A. D., 40
Aggressiveness, 141, 172, 173, 178
  in children with attention deficit–
    hyperactivity disorder, 146
Alexander, R. N., 14, 16, 17
Alexander, S. B., 14, 18, 21
Allen, E. M., 134
Allen, R. P., 14, 15, 17
Andrews, D. A., 78
Anesko, K. M., 15, 53
Anger control, in adolescents, 150
Anxiety, 43
Assessment, behavioral, 45–59; see also
  Functional analysis

approaches to, 25–27
  in attention deficit–hyperactivity dis-
    order, 44, 146–148
  in case illustrations, 159, 160, 164, 165,
    168, 169, 177, 179
  curriculum-based, 34
  direct, 33–35
  idiographic, 27, 28, 32, 33, 44
  in treatment, 49, 50, 59
Assessment funnel, 28–29
Atkeson, B. M., 7, 21, 22
Atkins, M. S., 53, 54
Attention deficit–hyperactivity disorder
  (ADHD), 27, 32, 43, 44, 145–148
  in case illustration, 158–163
  diagnosis of, 145, 146
  medication for, 147
  and response cost, 146, 151
  school–home notes with, 146–148,
    151
  screening for, 53, 54, 173
  treatment of, 44, 146, 147
Ayllon, T., 12, 13, 15, 17, 19, 22
Azrin, N. H., 141

Baer, D. M., 11, 30, 40
Bailey, J. S., 15, 17, 19, 20, 22
Barkley, R. A., 44, 53, 145
Bartlett, B. J., 34
Barton, E. S., 11, 12, 21
Bechtel, D. R., 140–142
Beck, A. T., 52–54
Beck, S., 11
Beck Depression Inventory (BDI), 52, 54
Behavior analysis, 29–33, 59
  model, 30, 32

Behavior maintenance techniques, 21, 22
Behavior modification, 10, 11, 18, 112,
 113, 177
 in children with attention deficit–
 hyperactivity disorder, 147
 negotiating, 84–96
Behavior Problem Checklist, 53
Beliefs, of teachers, 38
Bergan, J., 46, 49–51, 70
Bernal, M. E., 11
Berowitz, B. P., 11
Bijou, S. W., 30
Blechman, E. A., 12–16, 19, 20, 24
Bostow, E., 14, 18, 21
Bradford, D. C., 25
"Brag Sheet," 12, 14
Brody, G., 40
Broughton, S. F., 12, 13, 21
Buckholdt, D., 15
Budd, K. S., 12–15, 17, 18, 20
Buss, R. R., 52
Butler, J. F., 141

Candee, B. L., 141
Carey, M. P., 52, 55
Carper, L. B., 7, 40, 54, 55n
Case illustrations, 2, 3, 99–101, 109,
 134–136, 158–181
Cavell, T. A., 55
Chamberlain, P., 11
Checklists; *see* Questionnaires
Child Behavior Checklist (CBCL), 51, 52,
 160, 178
 Parent Report, 53
 Teacher Report, 53
 Youth Self-Report, 51, 52, 55
Child Intake Form for Use in a Parent
 Interview, 60–63
Child self-report instruments, 52
Children's Depression Inventory (CDI),
 52
 Parent's Version, 53
Clark, J. H., 35
Classroom behavior problems; *see* Disrup-
 tive behavior
Classroom environment, 35
Coats, K. I., 52
Coding systems, 56, 57
Communication
 case example, 2, 3
 guidelines for, 87, 94
 obstacles to, 3, 4
 parent–adolescent, 150
 partial, 14
 and school–home notes, 7, 23, 66
Compliance, 57, 173, 174

Conderman, L., 11
Conflict Behavior Questionnaire, 52, 53
Conners, C. K., 53, 54
Conners Parent Rating Scale (CPRS), 53
Conners Parent and Teacher Rating
 Scale, 53, 54, 178
Conners Teacher Rating Scale (CTRS),
 53, 54
Consistency, in work performance, 95
Contingency contract, 20, 91, 96, 180
 minimum time for, 96
 monitoring changes in, 103, 104
Contingency management, 10, 11, 44, 65,
 66, 166, 167
 with attention deficit–hyperactivity dis-
 order, 146
 goals in, 16
 home-based, 23; *see also* Reinforcement
Corbett, T. F., 14, 16, 17
Cranston, S., 134
Cristler, C., 134
Criterion-referenced tests, 34, 59
Cross-situational problems, 44
Curtis, M. J., 28

Data collection, 45–49, 71, 117, 118, 175
Davis, C. J., 45–51
Depression, 43
 assessment of, 52–55
 in children, 45
 in mothers, 40
Dietz, A., 56
Differential attention, 11
Discipline, 41, 42, 173
Disruptive behavior, 32
 consequences of, 17, 18
 monitoring, 56
 overcorrection for, 141
 and response cost, 134
 treatment for, 44
Dougherty, A., 14–16, 19–21
Dougherty, E. H., 14–16, 19–21
Drabman, R. S., 30
Dumas, J. E., 40
Dyadic Adjustment Scale, 54

Edelbrock, C., 51–55, 160
Elliott, S. N., 21–23, 28, 47, 52–54, 76,
 134
Embry, L. H., 40
Encopresis, 141
Enuresis, 141
Environment, and behavior, 31, 35
Enyart, P., 52, 53
Erbaugh, J., 52, 54

Essay writing, 142, 143
Evans, S., 52
Eyberg, S. M., 51, 53, 54
Eyberg Child Behavior Inventory (ECBI),
    51, 53

Fading procedures, 21, 22, 72, 110, 118,
    167
Families
    demographic variables of, 39
    dysfunction in, 8, 39, 42, 43
    screening for problems in, 55
Family Environment Scale, 54
Fathers, 42, 43, 164, 168
Feedback, 12, 13, 106, 112, 161
    to adolescents, 149, 151
    in attention deficit–hyperactivity dis-
        order, 147
    to children, 6, 7, 35, 37, 98, 99, 101,
        103, 112, 117, 118
    fading of, 110, 111
    to parents, 3, 7, 13, 24, 138, 179
    from peer tutor, 166
    positive, 12, 14
    and response cost, 138
    through school–home notes, 7, 72,
        106, 161, 174, 181
    self-, 58
    to teachers, 7, 84
Feld, J. K., 46, 51
Ferritor, D. E., 15
Forehand, R., 7, 11, 21, 22, 40, 57
Forgery, in notes, 84, 142
Foster, S. L., 52, 53, 91, 93, 94
Fox, J. J., 11
Foxx, R. M., 11, 140–142
Frangia, G. W., 11
Frentz, C., 134
Fuchs, C. S., 34
Fuchs, D., 34
Functional analysis, 32, 31, 59
    of academic skills deficits, 34
    collecting data for, 45, 46; see also In-
        terviewing
Funderburk, B. W., 54
Furey, W., 40

Gadow, K. D., 44
Gallimore, R., 16
Galvin, G., 134
Garber, S., 12, 13, 17–19, 22
Goldfarb, A. L., 12–15, 17, 18, 20
"Good behavior" letter, 13, 14, 17
"Good News Note," 19
Goyette, C. H., 53, 54

Graziano, A. M., 11
Gresham, F. M., 21, 28, 45–54, 76
Guidance counselors, 73, 164
Guidubaldi, J., 11
Gutkin, T. B., 28, 35
Guyer, B. D., 15

Hall, R. V., 134
Hamblin, R. L., 15
Hamerlynck, L. A., 11
Handy, L. C., 11
Happy face; see Response cost
Happy Note, 67, 127
Harris, D. B., 52
Hartmann, D. P., 25
Hawryluk, M. K., 35, 37
Heaton, R. C., 14, 15, 17
Herbert-Jackson, E., 11
Heffer, R. W., 55, 134
Hoge, R. D., 78
Hohman, R. J., 141
Home Situations Questionnaire, 53
Home-Based Rewards for Classroom Be-
    havior: Use of School–Home Notes,
    70–72, 115–118
Homework, 3, 42, 51, 57, 83, 84, 95
    in case illustration, 164–166
Homework Problem Checklist, 53
Horne, A. M., 141
House, A. E., 57
Hovell, M. F., 7, 12–14, 16, 18–22
Hsu, T., 141
Hyperactivity; see Attention deficit–
    hyperactivity disorder

Idiographic assessment, 27, 28, 32,
    33
    in attention deficit–hyperactivity dis-
        order, 27, 28
Ignoring, 11, 23
Imber, R. B., 14, 15, 17, 22
Imber, S. C., 14, 15, 17, 22
Inattentiveness, 160, 161, 163–165
Interviewing, 8, 36, 164, 165, 168, 169,
    177, 178
    in attention deficit–hyperactivity dis-
        order, 159
    behavioral, 45–51, 59
    behaviors, 48
    in depression, 45
    for problem analysis, 49, 59
    for problem evaluation, 49–50, 59
    for problem identification, 46, 47, 49,
        59
Issues Checklist, 52, 53

Jones, J. R., 11, 141

Karraker, R. J., 12, 13, 16, 17, 19
Kass, R. E., 56
Kelley, M. L., 7, 30, 40, 52, 54, 134, 158
Kendell, Ginger K., 92, 158
Kendell, H. J., 15
Kent, R. N., 52, 53
KeyMath Diagnostic Test, 34
King, H. E., 11
Kirby, F. D., 15
Kleinert, M. D., 11
Knowledgeability, of teachers, 35, 37
Kotanchik, N. L., 12–14, 19
Kovacs, M., 52, 53
Kramer, J. J., 28, 76
Kratochwill, T. R., 27, 36, 47, 48

Lahey, B. B., 12, 14–16, 19–22, 44
Layman, D., 15
Learning disability, 177, 181
Leibowitz, J. M., 12–15, 17, 18, 20
Lemanek, K. L., 21
Lentz, F. E., Jr., 25, 34–36, 56
Little, L. M., 134
Long, J. D., 11

MacDonald, G., 16
MacDonald, W. S., 16
MacPherson, E. M., 141
Madsen, C. H., 14, 15, 18, 19, 21
Marital conflict, 31, 40, 168, 171
  and discipline problems, 169, 173
Martens, B. K., 21, 23, 55
Mash, E. J., 11, 55
Maternal dysfunction, 8, 31, 40
Matson, J. L., 141
McAllister, L. W., 11
McMahon, R. J., 57
Mendelson, N. M., 52, 54
Meuser, S. T., 141
Meyerrose, M., 134
Miller, Debbie, 158
Mindell, C., 12–15, 17, 18, 20
Mock, J., 52, 54
Monitoring
  of child's behavior, 20, 21, 56, 104
  of parents, 103
  of teacher, 57
Moos, B. S., 54
Moos, R. H., 54
Morales, R. G., 141
Moreland, F. R., 11

Mothers, 168, 169; *see also* Maternal dysfunction
Mothers' Activity Checklist, 54
Multidimensional Self-Concept Scale, 52
Murphy, H. A., 53, 54

Negotiation, 84–96
  of performance goals, 91
Norm-referenced tests, 34, 44

Observation
  in behavior analysis, 30
  in classroom, 55–57, 59, 160, 169, 178, 179
  coding in, 56, 57
  direct, 25, 44, 55–57, 59
  in home setting, 57
O'Dell, S. L., 11
O'Leary, K. D., 52, 53, 56
O'Leary, S. G., 15, 53
Ollendick, D. G., 141
Ollendick, T. H., 141
On-task/off-task behavior, 56, 57, 163, 178, 179
Oppositional behavior, 168, 169, 173
Ora, J. D., 11
Organizational skills, building, 148
Overcorrection, 11, 140–145, 179, 180
  characteristics of, 141, 142
  definition of, 140
  educational function of, 142
  forms of, 140, 141
  in school–home note program, 142–144
Owen, P. P., 11, 12, 21

Paper-and-pencil instruments, 51–55, 59
Parent report instruments, 53, 54
Parent training, 10, 18–20, 24
  in behavior management techniques, 18
Parent–child interactions, 41, 42, 44
Parent–teacher conference, 114
Parents
  cooperation of, in school–home note program, 68, 69, 73
  educational background of, 39
  expectations of, 40, 41
  handouts for, 70–72, 75, 115–118, 131, 132, 152–154, 175
  and negotiation for behavior change, 84, 86
  skills of, 41, 42
Patterson, G. R., 11
Pazulinec, P., 134

Peer interaction, 172
  negative, 31, 32, 173
Peer tutoring, 165–167
Pelham, W. E., 53, 54
Performance criteria, 95, 96, 175
  and point loss, 136
Peterson, R., 134
Phillips, E. L., 15, 17, 19, 20, 22
Piers, E. V., 52
Piers-Harris Children's Self-Concept
  Scale, 52
Piersel, W. C., 28
Pisor, K., 12, 13, 17–19, 22
Points, in response cost, 134–140, 153,
  154
  bankruptcy, 140
  techniques for taking away, 136, 137,
    153, 154
Porterfield, J. K., 11
Positive practice, 140–145, 150, 151, 180
Prinz, R. J., 52, 53
Praise, 11, 16, 23, 68, 90, 102, 161, 180
  from parents, 103
  plus privileges/rewards, 16, 17
  in response cost, 137, 138, 152, 153
  from teachers, 17, 101, 112, 139
Prinz, R. J., 52, 53
Privileges; *see* Rewards
Problem analysis, goals of, 49
Problem evaluation, 49, 50
  objectives of, 50
Problem identification interview, 46–51
  components of, 47
Problem solving, 7, 20, 94, 112
  and behavioral assessment, 27–29, 45–
    58
  collaborative, 23, 24
  evaluation of, 95, 96
  in response cost, 138, 139
  seven-step process of, 28
  teachers' skills in, 37
  team approach to, 69
  training in, 150
Prumo, F. M., 14, 15, 17
Public Law, 94-142, 1, 69
Public Law 99-457, 1
Punishment, 31, 89–91, 150, 151
  essay writing as, 142, 143
  guidelines for, 90, 118
  loss of privileges as, 89
  overcorrection as, 144, 145
  physical, 2, 90
  response cost as, 133, 152
  for tantrum behavior, 141

Quay, H. C., 52
Questionnaires, 51–55, 160, 178

child self-report, 52
parent report, 53, 54
teacher report, 54

Rapport, M. D., 147
Redd, W. H., 30
Reid, J. B., 11
Reinforcement, 14, 31
  and academic skills, 34, 35
  of appropriate behavior, 16, 32, 169,
    174
  delayed, 8
  follow-up on, 22
  home-based vs. school-based, 8, 14, 17,
    18, 23, 69
  negative, 31, 169, 170
  positive; *see* Rewards
  removal of, 133, 134
  teacher training in, 21
  and use of Star Charts, 132
Reisinger, J. J., 11
Report cards, 149
  daily, 4, 16, 21, 64; *see also* School–
    home note program
  and self-monitoring, 58
Response cost, 11, 16–18, 23, 133–140,
  150, 151
  considerations for using, 139, 140
  definition of, 133, 134, 152
  goal achievement in, 137, 138, 152,
    161–163
  instructions for using, 152–154
  in school–home note program, 134–
    136, 155, 156
  side effects of, 140
  types of, 134
  with younger children, 138, 153
Responsibility, training for in children,
  97, 98
Restitution, 140, 141, 180
  vs. positive practice, 142
Revised Children's Manifest Anxiety
  Scale, 52
Rewards, 16, 17, 86–96, 112, 117, 166,
  175
  age-related, 88, 150
  changes in, 103, 104
  vs. overcorrection, 145
  requirements for, 86
  in response cost, 153, 162
  selection of, 84, 86
  with use of monitoring chart, 180
  with use of Star Chart, 132, 171
Reynolds, C. R., 52
Reynolds, W. M., 52
Reynolds Adolescent Depression Scale, 52

Richmond, B. O., 52
Riner, L. S., 12–15, 17, 18, 20
Risley, T. R., 11
Ritalin, 147, 177
Robin, A. L., 91, 93, 94
Robinson, E. A., 51, 53
Role play, 144
Romanczyk, R. G., 56
Roper, B. L., 25
Ross, A. W., 51, 53
Rothstein, C., 14, 15, 17, 22
Rusch, F. R., 30

Safer, D. J., 14, 15, 17
Sajwaj, T., 134
Salend, S. J., 134
Sanctions; *see* Punishment
Santogrossi, D., 56
Saudargas, R. A., 14, 15, 18, 19, 21
Schaughency, E. A., 44
School personnel, 73
School records, 58, 59
School–home note monitoring chart,
    180, 181
School–home note program, 4–8
  administration of, 97–112
  advantages of, 7, 23, 24, 151
  and age/grade levels, 14, 67, 83
  appropriate clients for, 66–68, 112
  in case illustrations, 160–163, 165–
      168, 170–172, 174–176, 179–181
  contract in, 129, 130
  designing, steps in, 71, 72, 75, 84, 112,
      114, 115
  evaluation of, 104–110
  examples of notes, 5, 6, 74, 82, 83, 85,
      100, 120–126, 135, 155–157
  handouts for, 70–72, 75, 115–118
  introducing the concept of, 69–72
  minimum time for, 106
  obstacles to, 108
  with response-cost component, 155,
      156
  selecting team members for, 72
  side effects of, 109, 110
  social validity of, 22–24, 108
  with special populations, 145–148
Schrader, S. M., 13–16, 19, 20, 24
Schultz, L. A., 11
Schumacher, J. B., 7, 12–14, 16, 18–22
Schwebel, A. T., 11
Scott, J. W., 14, 15, 18, 19, 21
Scott, O., 52
Scott, R. B., 14, 18, 21
Self-esteem, 8, 159
Self-evaluation, 137, 139, 141

Self-monitoring, 58, 111
Self-talk, 32
Setting events, 31, 32, 160
  in behavior analysis, 30
Shapiro, E. S., 25, 27, 34–36, 47, 48, 56,
    58
Sherman, J. A., 7, 12–14, 16, 18–22
Shields, F., 15
Shoiock, G., 53
Single parents, 39
Smallwood, D. L., 35, 37
Smigel, J., 14, 16, 17
Smith, K., 40
Smith, L., 15
SNAP, 53
Social skills, training in, 150
Social Skills Rating System, 52–54
Social validity, of school–home notes,
    22–24, 108
Spanier, G. B., 54
Spanking, 2, 90
Special education, 177
Spinnato, N. C., 14, 15, 17
Spouse consistency, 73, 169
Sprague, R. S., 53
Stackowiak, J. G., 11
Stambaugh, E. E., 57
Star Chart, 131, 132, 171
Stone, C. A., 46, 51
Stress
  in mothers, 40
  in teachers, 38
Study skills, 150, 164–166
Stumphauzer, J. J., 11
Substance abuse, 42, 43
Sumner, J. H., 141
Suspension, from school, 18
Sutter–Eyberg Behavior Inventory, 54

Tantrum behavior, 141
Tardiness, 134
Target behaviors, 15, 16, 78–81, 92, 94,
    112
  checklist for, 105
  descriptors of, 80
  evaluation of, 108, 115
  identifying, 18, 78, 115, 116, 137, 174,
      175
Taylor, C. J., 12–16, 19, 20, 24
Teacher Interview for Academic Assess-
    ment, 36
Teacher report instruments, 54
Teachers
  and communication with parents, 1–4
  cooperativeness of with consultants, 35,
      38

monitoring of, 57
morale of, 38
reliability of, in monitoring, 20
and response-cost system, 134–136,
  153, 154
role of in school–home note program,
  97–99, 100–101
skills of, 37
training of in school–home note system, 21, 24, 181
variables affecting functioning of, 35,
  37, 38
Terdall, L. G., 55
Time management, 166
Time out, 11, 18, 23, 68
Todd, D. D., 14, 18, 21
Token economy, 12, 23, 66
Tombari, M., 46
Tourette syndrome, 176, 177, 181
Truancy, 17
Tucker, B., 134
Turco, T. L., 23

Ulrich, R. F., 53, 54

Wagner, R. F., 15
Wahler, R. G., 11, 31, 40, 57
Walker, J., 44
Ward, C., 52, 54
Wechsler, D., 160
Wechsler Intelligence Scale for Chil-
  dren—Revised (WISC-R), 160, 165,
  178
Weiner, H., 133, 134
Wells, R., 11
Werry, J. S., 53
Werry–Weiser–Peters Activity Rating
  Scale, 53
White, K. S., 53, 54
Williams, R. L., 11
Winett, R. A., 15
Winkler, R. C., 15
Witt, J. C., 21, 23, 28, 34, 47, 55, 76, 134
Wolf, M. M., 15, 17, 19, 20, 22